Should I
Eat the Yolk?

Should I Eat the Yolk?

SEPARATING FACTS FROM MYTHS TO GET YOU LEAN, FIT AND HEALTHY

JAMIE HALE

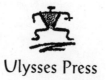

Ulysses Press

Published by:
ULYSSES PRESS
P.O. Box 3440
Berkeley, CA 94703
www.ulyssespress.com

ISBN: 978-1-56975-790-1
Library of Congress Control Number: 2009943777

Acquisitions Editor: Kelly Reed
Managing Editor: Claire Chun
Editor: Kathy Kaiser
Editorial staff: Lauren Harrison
Production: Judith Metzener
Index: Sayre Van Young
Front cover design: Double R Design
Front cover photo: ©istockphoto.com/AndrewJohnson
Back cover photos: ©shutterstock.com/Alaettin YILDIRIM, studio_chki, nimblewit

10 9 8 7 6 5 4 3 2 1

Printed in Canada by Webcom

Distributed by Publishers Group West

NOTE TO READERS
This book has been written and published strictly for informational purposes, and in no way should be used as a substitute for consultation with health-care professionals. You should not consider educational material herein to be the practice of medicine or to replace consultation with a physician or other medical practitioner. The author and publisher are providing you with information in this work so that you can have the knowledge and can choose, at your own risk, to act on that knowledge. The author and publisher also urge all readers to be aware of their health status and to consult health-care professionals before beginning any health program.

This book is dedicated to my wife, Brooke. You have been saying for years I need to write a book for the lay public. It's finally here. Enjoy.

CONTENTS

Acknowledgments   9

Introduction   11

Chapter 1 Health and Nutrition Claims   13

Chapter 2 Exercise Claims   62

Chapter 3 Finding the Right Diet for Weight Loss   107

References   114

Index   135

About the Author   144

ACKNOWLEDGMENTS

I would like to thank the HNE Research Group and all of my research associates for helping me gather the data that was necessary to write this book.

INTRODUCTION

Do I really need to drink 8 glasses of water a day?

Should I eat only low glycemic index carbohydrates when trying to lose weight?

Will heavy weight training make me bulky?

Should I eat the yolk?

These are just a few of the many questions that people interested in their health ask. With so much information available on health, exercise, and nutrition, finding the answers shouldn't be a problem. The information can be found in books, on the World Wide Web, and in the media. But with so much information out there and new facts coming out seemingly every week, the problem is sorting through it all and figuring out what is correct.

The first section of this book addresses health and nutrition claims. Each claim is presented in a question-and-answer format; this is followed by an investigation of the research on the subject. Here are some of the questions investigated: *Is bottled water safer to drink than tap water? Should food enjoyment be considered when dieting? Does eating specific types of foods together cause weight gain?* Many more questions are discussed.

The second section addresses exercise claims. These (and many other) questions are discussed: *Will exercise get rid of cellulite? Does heavy weight training decrease flexibility? Are certified fitness trainers highly qualified trainers?*

In the final section of the book, popular diet plans are analyzed, including the Atkins Diet, the South Beach Diet, Nutrisystem, the maple syrup diet (the diet that Beyoncé Knowles used to shed pounds for *Dreamgirls*), Weight Watchers, Jenny Craig, and many more. How nutritionally sound are these diets? Are any of them for you? Read the analysis and decide.

For much of my life, I have been involved with sports and fitness. At an early age, I received my first weight set and began participating in martial arts. In college, I was the founder and president of Eastern Kentucky University's boxing team. Shortly after graduating from college, I opened up the gym Total Body Fitness (one of the top 30 gyms in the country, according to *Men's Health*), which I owned and managed for eleven years before selling it in 2008.

While I owned Total Body Fitness, I competed as a bodybuilder, began my writing career, founded HNE Research Group (a group that analyzes and writes about scientific research), lectured about health and fitness, and continued to participate in martial arts. From my preteen years to the present day, I have had a passion for fitness and fitness education. Currently, I spend six to eight hours a day conducting research and another three to four hours designing fitness plans. My personal exercise regimen includes a wide array of activities: kayaking, weight training, kickboxing, skateboarding, and so on.

It was my never-ending quest for knowledge about fitness that led me to write this book.

CHAPTER 1

HEALTH AND NUTRITION CLAIMS

Do high insulin levels cause obesity?

ANSWER: Elevated insulin levels do not cause obesity. Obese people who eat excessive calories may also have high insulin levels. Do not mistake correlation for causation. Fat gain is the result of excessive calories.

INVESTIGATION: This subject has been misunderstood in the fitness industry for years. Many experts blame obesity on elevated insulin, but the scientific data do not support this claim. Insulin plays numerous roles in metabolism, but popular diet gurus generally have no idea of the complexity and the various effects that insulin has on the body.

Calorie restriction, independent of diet composition (for example, 15 percent to 73 percent carbohydrate) improves glycemic control (blood glucose control). "The ability to lose weight on a calorie restricted diet over a short-term period does not vary in obese healthy women as a function of insulin resistance (decreased ability of target tissues to respond properly to insulin) or hyperinsulinemia (high insulin levels)," says nutrition researcher M. R. Freedman.

A review by Freedman, published in *Obesity Research*, in March 2001, reported that subjects consuming 1,000-calorie diets containing 15 percent carbohydrate had significantly lower insulin levels compared with those consuming 1,000-calorie diets containing 45 percent carbohydrate. Yet there was no difference in weight loss between the two groups. In the review, a study was cited where researchers studied 10 obese patients who were fed low-calorie (1,500 calories a day) liquid formula diets containing either 72 percent or 0 percent carbohydrate for four weeks before switching to the other diet. A significant reduction in insulin levels was noted when subjects consumed the formula containing 0 percent carbohydrate. Refeeding the high-carbohydrate formula resulted in a marked increase in insulin. However, patients lost 0.75 to 2.0 kg a week, irrespective of caloric distribution.

Recently, studies have shown that the selective genetic disruption of insulin signaling in the brain leads to increased food intake and obesity in animals. This demonstrates that intact insulin signaling in the central nervous system is required for normal body weight regulation.

Is it all right to eat fruit when dieting?

ANSWER: Fruit is highly recommended while dieting. Fruit is low in calories, is nutrient dense, contains fiber, and can be very filling (particularly fruits that contain a fair amount of soluble fiber, for example, apples). In addition, fruit soothes the sweet tooth for many people.

INVESTIGATION: The fear of fruit comes from the relatively high sugar content in fruit and the potential for weight gain.

Some studies have suggested that 60 grams or more of fructose a day can stimulate de novo lipogenesis (the process whereby excessive carbohydrates are converted to triglycerides in the liver), increase blood triglycerides, and induce insulin resistance (decrease the ability of target tissues to respond properly to insulin). This could contribute to weight gain and health problems. But keep in mind that a piece of fruit generally contains only 6–7 grams of fructose. You would have to eat a very large amount of fruit to get 60 grams of fructose. In most studies, the high consumption of fructose is generally due to the consumption of high levels of high-fructose corn syrup. Another consideration is that fructose causes minimal insulin secretion. So even if fructose consumption was high enough to elevate fat synthesis, a lack of insulin would probably result in increased fat burning. Assuming a calorie deficit, it all evens itself out at the end of the day.

What about the sugar content of fruit? Isn't sugar a no-no when dieting? It's important to realize that there are various types of sugars. According to the Advanced Carbohydrate Classification System, sugars include glucose, fructose, galactose, sucrose, maltose, lactose, and a few others. Fruits contain glucose, fructose, and sucrose in varying degrees. Do these sugars contribute to obesity? They can contribute to obesity if you consume excessive amounts. But if eaten in moderation, they do not promote obesity.

Is bottled water safer to drink than tap water?

ANSWER: Many consider bottled water to be safer and purer than tap water. But my thorough analysis of a massive amount of scientific research and other sources of data did not lead me to believe that bottled water was any safer than tap water. The biggest advantage of bottled water is the convenience of the container.

INVESTIGATION: A study conducted in Ohio in 2000 looked at the fluoride level and bacterial content of commercially bottled waters versus municipal tap water. Fifty-seven samples of five categories of bottled water were purchased from local stores. Samples of tap water were collected in sterile containers from the four local water-processing plants. Fluoride levels within the range recommended for drinking water by the Ohio Environmental Protection Agency were found in only three samples of bottled water tested.

The fluoride levels of tap water samples were within 0.04 mg/L of the optimal fluoride level of 1.00 mg/L. The bacterial counts, or bacterial colony-forming units (CFUs), in the bottled water samples ranged from less than 0.01 CFU/mL to 4,900 CFUs/mL. In contrast, bacterial counts in samples of tap water ranged from 0.2 to 2.7 CFUs/mL.

Of the bottled water purchased in Cleveland, only 5 percent fell within the required fluoride range recommended by the state, compared with 100 percent of the tap water samples. The researchers concluded that, when measured by these standards, bottled water was less pure than tap water.

The Natural Resources Defense Council (NRDC) published the results of a four-year study in which they tested more than 1,000 samples of 103 brands of bottled water. The study indicated that approximately 25 percent or more of bottled water was really just tap water. The NRDC also found that 18 of the 103 brands tested had more bacteria than allowed under microbiological purity guidelines. About one-fifth of the waters contained synthetic organic chemicals, but these were generally at levels below state and federal standards.

Bottled water is subject to less-rigorous purity standards and less-frequent tests for bacterial and chemical contaminants than those required for tap water. Bottled water plants test for coliform bacteria once a week. In contrast, city tap water is tested 100 or more times a month for coliform bacteria.

Does bottled water taste better than tap water?

ANSWER: The results of most blind taste tests indicate no difference between the taste of tap water and that of bottled water. I have carried out my own blind taste tests, and my results have shown that there is no difference in taste. Interestingly, the results are different in nonblind taste tests.

INVESTIGATION: When blind tests are conducted, the taste buds really don't seem to think that bottled water tastes better than tap water. In 2001, ABC's *Good Morning America* conducted a blind water taste test. The viewers' preferences were as follows: 12 percent Evian, 19 percent O-2, 24 percent Poland Spring, and 45 percent New York City tap water. Yorkshire Water, the water department in Yorkshire, England, found that 60 percent of 2,800 people surveyed could not tell the difference between the local tap water and UK bottled water.

The hosts of Showtime's television series *Penn & Teller: Bullshit* conducted a blind taste test comparing waters. The test showed that 75 percent of New Yorkers preferred city tap water to bottled waters. The hosts of the show conducted another test in a trendy Southern California restaurant. A water sommelier handed out water menus with extravagant prices to the patrons. The patrons had no idea that all of the fancy bottles of water were filled with the same water from a water hose in the back of the restaurant. Patrons were willing to pay $7 a bottle for "L'eau du Robinet" (French for "tap water"), "Agua de Culo" (Spanish for "ass water"), and "Amazone" ("filtered through the Brazilian rainforest's natural filtration system").

Does it matter where calories come from? Or is a calorie a calorie, regardless of its source?

ANSWER: Technically, a calorie is a calorie. The definition of a calorie does not change, *but* different calorie sources have different properties and they affect the body in various ways. So when considering nutrient value, effects on appetite, intolerances, and allergies, there are differences in calorie sources.

Some low-carbohydrate enthusiasts claim that calories from fat are different from calories from carbohydrates. It is true that short-term weight loss is usually greater with a low-carbohydrate diet than a higher-carbohydrate diet, even when the calories are equal. This, however, is largely due to water loss.

INVESTIGATION: A calorie is a unit of energy. It is the amount of energy, or heat, that it takes to raise the temperature of 1 gram of water 1 degree Celsius (1.8 degrees Fahrenheit).

The energy derived from foods when they are oxidized in the body is measured in kilocalories (thousands of calories). A kilocalorie is the amount of energy required to raise 1,000 grams of water 1 degree Celsius. *Kilocalorie* is written as "Calorie" (with a capital C) or it may be abbreviated to "Kcalorie" or "Kcal." Therefore, whenever the word *calorie* is used in connection with food or nutrition, the meaning is always "kilocalorie" or "calorie."

In terms of fat loss, a low-calorie diet consisting of Twinkies will result in weight loss, just like a low-calorie diet consisting of fruits and vegetables will. When considering which is more nutritious, fruits and vegetables win, hands down. Which is more filling? Fruits and vegetables win again. When considering issues other than energy content, it's not just about calories. We get calories from four sources, including protein (4 Kcal per gram), fat (9 Kcal per gram), carbohydrate (4 Kcal per gram), and alcohol (7 Kcal per gram).

Are carbohydrates essential nutrients?

ANSWER: Carbohydrates are not classified as essential nutrients. This does not imply that they are not essential for health. They are essential for life, but it is not essential that they come from diet. Carbohydrates are not classified as essential nutrients because the body synthesizes glucose (which comes from carbohydrates) from noncarbohydrate sources.

INVESTIGATION: Essential nutrients must be obtained from diet because the body does not produce them, or at least does not provide them in adequate amounts. Essential nutrients include vitamins and minerals, essential fatty acids (Omega 3 and Omega 6), and essential amino acids. Nonessential nutrients are produced in adequate amounts by the body; therefore, it is not vital to obtain them through diet. Glucose is synthesized in the body from noncarbohydrate sources.

Can some people with lactose intolerance consume some dairy?

ANSWER: Not all individuals with lactose intolerance have to avoid dairy completely. Some can still ingest small amounts of dairy containing lactose. The proper treatment varies with the individual.

INVESTIGATION: Lactose intolerance (acquired lactase deficiency) is the most common form of carbohydrate intolerance. Lactase levels are high in neonates, permitting digestion of milk. In most ethnic groups (80 percent of African Americans and Hispanics and almost 100 percent of Asians), the levels decrease in the post-weaning period, rendering older children and adults unable to digest significant amounts of lactose. However, 80 to 85 percent of Caucasians from northwest European descent produce lactase throughout life and are thus able to digest milk and milk products.

Avoiding dairy products often treats lactose intolerance. However, because the degree of lactose mal-absorption varies greatly, many patients can ingest up to 12 ounces (18 grams of lactose) of milk daily without symptoms. In general, the 12 ounces should be divided up throughout the day. I have found that ingesting 4 ounces three times a day works well with most people. Yogurt is usually tolerated because it contains an appreciable amount of lactase produced by intrinsic *Lactobacilli*.

Lactose intolerance can also be treated by consuming lactose-free products or by adding a commercially prepared lactase to milk.

Should food enjoyment be considered when dieting?

ANSWER: Dieting doesn't have to be torture. Include foods in your diet that are enjoyable to help ensure dieting success. Just be sure not to go overboard with excessive calories. Overall nutrition should be a consideration as well.

INVESTIGATION: Common wisdom states, "If it tastes good, it's not good for you." It also says, "If you get to eat the foods you like, you're not dieting." There is no evidence to support these claims. In fact, many diets fail due to this attitude. When dieting, there is no reason that the foods have to be bland or taste bad. I knew a bodybuilder who used to mix tuna, water, and protein powder in a blender for lunch. His idea was that food didn't need to taste good; what really mattered was getting nutrients. That mentality may work for some. But if you tell the majority of people that their food must be dull or that they can't ever eat what they like, you are setting them up for failure. Flavor in the diet helps to ensure success, as long as the flavor is not pushing you over your calorie budget.

Given that coffee raises insulin levels acutely, should it be avoided?

ANSWER: Drinking coffee in moderation is fine, and according to recent studies, it may be beneficial for some with serious health problems. Those who are caffeine sensitive (and experience "jittery" side effects) should avoid coffee, however.

INVESTIGATION: Insulin is an essential hormone. It is needed for various purposes, including survival. It is not the villain that many would have you believe. Studies suggest that long-term caffeine ingestion actually lowers the risk of developing type 2 diabetes. In addition, some studies have found that coffee consumption lowers the risk of metabolic syndrome, and improves cardiovascular health. Caffeine increases the release of adrenaline, which, in turn, increases fat mobilization. Some athletes will, at times, use caffeine as a training aid and an appetite suppressant.

Does dietary fat have beneficial effects on testosterone levels?

ANSWER: Most studies show that the consumption of dietary fat increases total testosterone levels. Are elevated testosterone levels healthy? Slightly elevated levels may provide health benefits. Super-high levels for long periods of time, however, may be detrimental to health.

INVESTIGATION: A study published in 1984 in the *Journal of Steroid Biochemistry* examined the effects of dietary fat content and the ratio of polyunsaturated to saturated fatty acids (P/S ratio) on serum sex hormones in 30 healthy male volunteers. The customary diet of the subjects, which contained 40 percent fat, was replaced for a six-week period with a diet containing 15 percent fat and a higher P/S ratio. The calories of the diets were approximately the same. The results of the study indicated that in men a decrease in dietary fat content and an increase in the degree of polyunsaturated fatty acids reduced testosterone levels.

A study published in *Medicine and Science in Sports and Exercise* investigated serum sex hormones, including testosterone, after subjects ate either a lacto-ovo vegetarian diet or a mixed diet. The lacto-ovo diet resulted in lower total testosterone levels compared with the mixed diet. After six weeks on the diets, the total testosterone was significantly lower in subjects on the lacto-ovo diet during exercise than in subjects on the mixed diet.

Can people with hypothyroidism lose weight?

ANSWER: The road may be a little rockier, but with the right plan, people with hypothyroidism can lose weight. With this population, it is sometimes difficult to find a maintenance calorie level, as thyroid levels can vary greatly. Even if the maintenance level is found, it may change drastically over short periods of time. I have seen people with this disorder drop large amounts of weight. But in order to do this, they have to jump over the mental block of thinking, *I can't lose weight; I have a thyroid problem.*

INVESTIGATION: Hypothyroidism is a condition in which a person has low levels of thyroid hormone. With this condition, thyroxine levels drop and the body's metabolism slows down. Signs of hypothyroidism include weakness, constipation, fatigue, weight gain, joint or muscle pain, and depression.

It seems as though almost everyone who has a weight problem is convinced that he or she has hypothyroidism. This isn't usually the case. But even if you do have this condition, it doesn't mean that weight loss is impossible. If calorie intake is adjusted appropriately, weight loss is possible. If you consistently eat fewer calories than your maintenance level, you will lose weight. If you are consistently eating fewer calories than your maintenance requirement but you are *not* losing weight, you are miscounting your calories. If you have hypothyroidism, it may be harder for you to lose weight than others—but it can be done.

Does eating specific types of foods together cause weight gain?

ANSWER: Eating particular types of foods together does not cause weight gain unless their consumption results in a positive calorie balance. When you were first born, you may have drunk breast milk, a food containing fat, protein, and carbohydrate. Most of us have spent the majority of our lives eating a mixed diet. The anecdotal and scientific evidence refute the validity of the macronutrient food-combining theory.

INVESTIGATION: The claim that eating certain types of foods together results in weight gain is often perpetuated by supporters of the macronutrient food-combining theory. The theory says that carbohydrates shouldn't be mixed with protein/fat meals and fat shouldn't be mixed with protein/carbohydrate meals. The theory generally assumes that insulin and blood levels of fat should never be raised at the same time and that insulin is the key contributor to obesity.

A study published in 2000 in the *International Journal of Obesity* compared the weight loss of subjects eating low-calorie balanced diets with that of subjects eating low-calorie food-combining diets. The results indicated that there was no significant difference between these two groups in the amount of weight lost. In addition, a great deal of anecdotal evidence exists that denies the need for food combining. We have evolved on a mixed diet. However, food combining may be beneficial with regard to calorie control. You can go a long way in decreasing total caloric intake by eliminating an entire macronutrient from a meal.

Does eating grapefruit speed up fat loss?

ANSWER: Many competitive bodybuilders refuse to eat any fruit except grapefruit. They are under the impression that grapefruit, unlike other fruits, has special fat-burning properties. But although grapefruit is a nutritious food source, it is no better than other fruits when it comes to fat loss.

INVESTIGATION: Grapefruit fat loss proponents claim that naringin, a secondary plant metabolite that gives grapefruit its bitter taste, is a magic fat-burning agent. A study published in 2006 in *Clinical and Experimental Pharmacology* and *Physiology* found that naringin does not significantly alter calorie expenditure. The double-blind study measured calorie expenditure before and systematically for eight hours after a single dose of caffeine with and without naringin in ten apparently healthy individuals.

Nutritionist Alan Aragon said this in a 2009 online nutrition roundtable: "As far as grapefruit being a 'magic' fruit for dieters, recent research performed last year by Fujioka's team can be interpreted to indicate that possibility. But the big problem is that we're talking about 3.3 pounds more weight loss than the placebo over a 12-week period. Frankly, you can get that kind of weight loss by scratching your ass and singing in the shower. Instead of using apple juice as a placebo, I'd like to see them compare the effect of a range of whole fruits with grapefruit. Then you'll see the differences diminish into [even] less significance."

He added, "If the lunacy over grapefruit makes people consume fruit when they hadn't before (or makes them consume more fruit), then great. That's a positive. But I think folks need to be aware that grapefruit is one of the most medication-interactive foods out there. They should really do their investigating diligently if they're on any meds."

Do cortisol blockers, such as Relacore, cause weight loss?

ANSWER: Relacore does not cause weight loss. Like many other supplements, this product is overhyped. Its success can be attributed to the fancy rhetoric that appeals to people's emotions used by advertisers.

INVESTIGATION: Cortisol is secreted from the middle layer of the adrenal cortex. It is released in times of stress and does many things in the body, including divert glucose away from the muscles and toward the brain, facilitate the action of adrenaline hormones, and prevent the overreaction of the immune system to injury. It also is an anti-inflammatory, increases protein breakdown, and stimulates LPL, a fat storage enzyme. Some studies have shown a significant increase in protein breakdown following an acute elevation of cortisol, and a significant increase in body fat levels when cortisol reaches super-high levels.

Supplement Watch, a Web site providing commentary on the pros and cons of dietary supplementation, claims that magnolia bark, found in Relacore, decreases cortisol levels. But do decreases in cortisol mean weight loss? The majority of research shows that obese people have normal cortisol levels. A study published in 1986 in *Psychiatry Research* found elevated cortisol levels in healthy, starving (meaning, not absorbing dietary nutrients, which in many cases improves health parameters, especially in chronically obese people) women who had lost weight. Not what you would expect to find if the hormone really causes weight gain!

Are high-protein diets bad for bone health?

ANSWER: A high-protein diet that lacks sufficient amounts of calcium and Vitamin D may cause harm to bones. But a high-protein diet that contains sufficient amounts of calcium and Vitamin D can have positive effects on bone health.

INVESTIGATION: You have probably heard the claim that high-protein diets are bad for bones because they cause calcium loss. However, when examining the scientific evidence, we see a different picture. A large study published in the *Journal of Bone and Mineral Research*, in 2000, showed that elderly men and women who consumed the most animal protein had the lowest rate of bone loss, whereas those who consumed little protein had much higher rates of bone loss.

Another study, this one published in the *American Journal of Clinical Nutrition*, in 1999, showed that postmenopausal women who consumed the highest amount of protein—particularly animal protein—were the least likely to have experienced hip fractures and had the strongest bones. In 1982, a study published in the *Journal of Laboratory and Clinical Medicine* showed that in free-living (meaning uncontrolled, or lacking supervision) middle-aged women—who were studied in a metabolic ward and ate diets that matched their everyday intakes of protein and phosphorus—calcium losses were significantly positively correlated with protein intake. Calcium balance was significantly negatively correlated with protein intake. This study, which has been cited extensively, has contributed to the common belief that protein is harmful to bone. Almost two decades later, in an editorial that was featured in the *American Journal of Clinical Nutrition*, Robert Heaney (the researcher) critiqued his own study and reported on recent findings.

Heaney said this: "[An] analysis of the diets of hunter-gatherer societies, and [that of] nitrogen isotope ratios of fossil bone collagen, indicate that human physiology evolved in the context of diets with high amounts of animal protein. Although caution has been urged in the interpretation of such analyses, it remains true that there is certainly no evidence that primitive humans had low intakes of either total protein or animal protein. That, coupled with the generally very robust skeletons of our hominid forbears, makes it difficult to sustain a case, either evidential or deductive, for overall skeletal harm related either to protein intake or to animal protein. Indeed, the balance of the evidence seems to indicate the opposite."

Research suggests that high-protein diets that include sufficient amounts of calcium and vitamin D do not negatively affect bone health. Researchers at Tufts University in Boston found that adequate ingestion of dietary calcium helps to promote a positive effect of dietary protein on the skeletons of older adults. Also, phosphorus (found, for example, in milk and meat) and potassium (found, for example, in milk, legumes, and grains) reduce calcium loss, helping to negate any protein-induced urinary calcium excretion.

Do high-protein diets increase the risk of coronary heart disease (CHD)?

ANSWER: High-protein diets that contain excessive calories and are high in fat may increase the risk factors associated with coronary heart disease (CHD). But high-protein diets that are low to moderate in calories and saturated fat do not increase those risk factors. I generally recommend a few servings of lean red meat each week. Red meat is loaded with micronutrients and is a good source of high-quality protein.

INVESTIGATION: A review published in 2005 in *Asia Pacific Journal of Clinical Nutrition* looked at the relationship between red meat consumption and CHD factors. Fifty-four studies were reviewed.

Here is one finding of the review: "Substantial evidence from recent studies shows that lean red meat trimmed of visible fat does not raise total blood cholesterol and LDL-cholesterol levels." This is another finding: "[L]ean red meat is low in saturated fat, and if consumed in a diet low in SFA [saturated fatty acids], is associated with reductions in LDL-cholesterol in both healthy and hypercholesterolemia [high-cholesterol] subjects." And here is one more finding of the review: "[L]ean red meat trimmed of visible fat, which is consumed in a diet low in saturated fat does not increase cardiovascular risk factors."

Are high-protein diets bad for the kidneys?

ANSWER: Research indicates that there is no evidence that a high intake of protein causes kidney damage in healthy individuals.

INVESTIGATION: The media often report that large amounts of protein stress the kidneys. Indeed, protein restriction is a common treatment for people with kidney problems. What does science say about the claim that a high-protein diet has a negative effect on the kidneys? A review published in 2005 in *Nutrition and Metabolism* investigated the available evidence regarding the effects of protein intake on kidney function, with a particular emphasis on kidney disease. Here is what the researchers found: "Although excessive protein intake remains a health concern in individuals with preexisting renal disease, the literature lacks significant research demonstrating a link between protein intake and the initiation or progression of renal disease in healthy individuals....[A]t present, there is not sufficient proof to warrant public health directives aimed at restricting dietary protein intake in healthy adults for the purpose of preserving renal function."

Should I eat only low glycemic index carbohydrates when trying to lose weight?

ANSWER: The bulk of the evidence suggests that glycemic index (GI) has no significant effect on weight loss, so low GI diets are not superior to high GI diets. Some studies indicate that people eat less when consuming low GI diets, while others indicate no such difference between the two. Regardless of GI content, other factors must be considered when looking at a comprehensive nutrition program. Low GI diets generally have fewer calories and are more nutritious. The GI of a food is altered when a person consumes that food with other foods. A food's GI can even be affected by a person's previous meals. In most cases, the GI of a food is more important if an individual has metabolic abnormalities relating to blood glucose and insulin (for example, type 2 diabetes, insulin resistance, or metabolic syndrome).

INVESTIGATION: The glycemic index (GI) is a ranking of carbohydrate foods and their immediate impact on blood glucose levels. All foods are compared with a reference food, such as pure glucose, in equivalent carbohydrate amounts. Foods ranking high on the index are often called "bad carbs"; foods ranking low are called "good carbs." However, Professors David Jenkins and Tom Wolever, the creators of the glycemic index, never used the terms "bad carbs" and "good carbs." Nutritionists, many of whom have misused the GI to promote their services, created the terminology.

A study published in 2005 in the *Journal of Nutrition* investigated the effects of reduced GI and glycemic loads on weight loss and insulin sensitivity in obese men and women. Obese subjects were assigned to one of three groups: a high-fat diet, a high GI diet, or a low GI diet. There was no significance difference in weight loss among the groups. A research review published in 2002 in *Obesity Review* analyzed studies comparing the effects of high and low GI foods. Anne Raben, the researcher, concluded that "there is no evidence at present that low GI foods are superior to high GI foods in regards to long-term body weight control."

In an interview published at MaxCondition.com in 2009, nutritionist Alan Aragon had this to say about the GI: "In the vast majority of trials lasting 6 months or longer, GI has no significant effect on bodyweight or body composition."

To maximize weight loss, should I eat small amounts every two to three hours?

ANSWER: Generally, I suggest that my clients eat three to five times a day. As long as macronutrients (protein, fat, and carbohydrate) and energy intake are equal, meal frequency does not significantly affect the outcome. Of course, personal preference should be considered. If you like to eat more often, that's fine. On another note, some studies have suggested that if protein intake is too low, eating more frequently might help to prevent protein loss.

INVESTIGATION: When I was a competitive boxer and seriously involved in mixed martial arts, I ate two meals a day. At the height of my bodybuilding career, when I was my heaviest, I was eating seven times a day. When I was at my leanest and following the XDL (Xtreme Density and Leanness) diet, I was eating four or five very low-calorie meals a day. As far as being mentally alert or feeling good, I really couldn't see much difference between two meals and five meals a day. When I ate seven times a day, I was eating a ton of calories and really didn't feel very well most of the time.

A research review published in 1997 in the *British Journal of Nutrition* investigated the possibility that eating frequently might prevent obesity. When the researchers reviewed studies that measured twenty-four-hour energy expenditure (calorie expenditure), they found no difference between nibbling (frequent eating) and gorging (eating big meals less often). In addition, the researchers found that, with the exception of a single study, there was no evidence that weight loss on low-calorie regimens was altered by meal frequency. A study published in 1987 in *Annals of Nutrition and Metabolism* compared the effects of one meal versus five meals a day. Changes in body weight weren't statistically significant. Urinary nitrogen excretion was slightly greater with a single daily meal, indicating that the number of meals a day influenced protein metabolism.

In other words, there was a slightly greater loss in protein when consuming a single meal daily. The results of the study demonstrated that the meal frequency did not influence energy balance. When considering meal frequency for individuals with metabolic disorders, more-frequent meals may be beneficial. David Jenkins, cocreator of the glycemic index, has suggested that more-frequent meals help individuals with type 2 diabetes and hyperlipidemia (high levels of fat in the blood) deal with the rate of glucose absorption and elevated insulin responses.

Are dietary supplements necessary?

ANSWER: If you are getting enough nutrients from your food, you don't need supplements, although at times supplementing is more convenient and, in some cases, cheaper. Supplements have been used as a successful training aid in many programs. And some people prefer to get their nutrients in the form of a pill or powder, while others prefer whole foods. Either can work. Just be sure you get your nutrients.

INVESTIGATION: Do you really need to spend hundreds of dollars a month on supplements if your nutritional practices are optimal? No, you don't. Dietary supplements were originally intended to supplement the training and nutrition program, not replace it. Today, supplements are often given priority over training and nutrition. It seems as though almost everyone is using them, including the muscular employees at the local supplement shop, the big guys at the gym, models, actors, athletes, and older adults. The subjects of training and nutrition might never arise when you discuss supplements with a salesperson. "Gain 10 pounds in one week!" "Add 40 pounds to your bench in a month!" Those are the types of claims many supplement companies make. They are making the oldest type of marketing pitch in the world: an appeal to the emotions.

In an article published in *Clinics in Sport Medicine*, in 2007, well-respected protein researcher Kevin Tipton said, "There is no reason to recommend protein supplements per se because there is no evidence that supplements work better than foods."

Before you purchase a supplement, ask to see scientific articles or research that supports the supplement's claims. Be critical of the data, especially when the company selling the product funds the publication of the data.

Is it okay to eat dairy when trying to lose weight?

ANSWER: Dairy products are nutritious and help to build strong bones and muscles. A typical serving of dairy contains 80 to 150 calories. If you are trying to lose weight, low-fat dairy is recommended. The low-fat versions are significantly lower in calories. When consuming dairy, if you experience bloating or an upset stomach, try taking lactase pills, switching dairy sources, eating smaller amounts, or consuming dairy foods in the same meal with nondairy foods. Of course, if you have a dairy allergy, avoid dairy.

INVESTIGATION: Dairy products are rich in protein, calcium, and various other nutrients. Most randomized, controlled studies have shown that milk consumption benefits those looking to build bone and muscle strength. Still, vegan groups try to convince people that dairy is bad for their health. This is true only for people who are allergic to dairy (although research indicates that true

31

dairy allergies are very rare) or who can't digest dairy. In those cases, dairy should be avoided. The digestion problem is often due to lactose intolerance.

Are low-carbohydrate diets bad for the brain?

ANSWER: Low-carbohydrate diets (ketogenic diets) have been used as treatment for a wide array of disorders. At this point, evidence does not suggest that ketogenic diets are harmful to the brain. However, more long-term research needs to be conducted in this area. Ketogenic diets work well for some people, although they are hell for others. If you feel unwell while following the diet, switch diets. There are many diet plans that lead to weight loss.

INVESTIGATION: Low-carbohydrate diets (ketogenic diets) promote the increased use of ketone bodies (a fuel substance that can be used by most of the body as a substitute for glucose) which can be used by the brain. Is this safe for the brain? An examination of epileptic children who follow a ketogenic diet and spend years in ketosis revealed no negative effects on cognitive function, except fatigue in the beginning stages of the diet.

Low-carbohydrate diets are used as treatment for some diseases. An article published in 2003 in *Universitats-Kinderklinik Essen* (a journal from a German university) reported that low-carbohydrate diets have been used for decades to treat intractable childhood epileptics, but they can also be used for treating deficiencies in transporting glucose from the blood (for example, glucose transporter type 1 deficiency syndrome) and treating abnormally high lactic acid levels caused by an enzyme deficiency (pyruvate dehydrogenase complex deficiency).

A study published in 2004 in *Neurobiology of Aging* suggests that beta-hydroxybutyrate (a ketone body) may improve cognitive functioning in older adults with memory disorders, such as Alzheimer's disease and mild cognitive disorders. Furthermore, in a review published in 2004 in *Prostaglandins,*

Leukotrienes and Essential Fatty Acids, the researcher noted, "Mild ketosis may offer therapeutic potential in a variety of different common and rare disease states." These disease states include those due to insulin resistance or substrate insufficiencies (the inability of enzymes to act on fats, proteins and so on), those due to free radical damage (unstable high-energy particles that can cause damage to the body), and those due to hypoxia (low oxygen levels in the blood and bodily tissues). Some studies have also shown that ketogenic diets can be used in the treatment of Parkinson's disease and brain tumors.

Do low-carbohydrate diets lead to weight loss?

ANSWER: Low-carbohydrate diets that result in significant weight and fat loss are low in calories. When severely limiting carbohydrates, a big drop in calories is to be expected. However, some individuals will compensate for the carbohydrate reduction by consuming more fat. If the increased fat consumption leads to excessive calories, body weight will increase. The metabolic advantage that low-carbohydrate diet proponents support is fiction, and has been soundly refuted by scientific evidence.

INVESTIGATION: If you eat only a small amount of carbohydrates, you can eat all the protein and fat you like and still lose weight—or so low-carbohydrate diet advocates say. Robert Atkins, MD, claims that his low-carbohydrate diet yields "metabolic advantages that will allow overweight individuals to eat as many or more calories as they were eating before starting the diet yet still lose pounds and inches," as reported by M. R. Freedman, nutrition researcher, in *Obesity Research*. Science, however, does not support this claim. Atkins cites studies to support his claim of the metabolic advantage offered by low-carbohydrate dieting. Yet the studies he cites actually *refute* the notion of this metabolic advantage. In one of the studies, obese individuals confined to a metabolic ward were given diets with the same ratio of fat, protein, and carbohydrate, but different amounts of calories. Individuals who ate the least amount of calories lost the most weight.

In another study, 14 obese patients were fed 1,000-calorie diets that were either 90 percent protein, 90 percent fat, or 90 percent carbohydrate. Each subject followed one of the three diets for five to nine days before being switched to another diet. Twenty-one days later, all the patients had lost weight. However, patients consuming 90 percent fat lost the most weight over five to nine days, which can be explained by changes in water balance, whereas those consuming 90 percent carbohydrate lost little to no weight in five to nine days.

In a study published in 1990 in the *Journal of the American Dietetic Association*, researcher Betty Alford and colleagues concluded, "[T]here is no statistically significant effect derived in an overweight adult female population from manipulation of percentage of carbohydrate in a 1,200-Kcal diet. Weight loss is the result of reduction in caloric intake in proportion to caloric requirements."

Are the Recommended Dietary Allowances (RDA) protein guidelines sufficient for athletes?

ANSWER: RDA guidelines are not sufficient for athletes. The information presented in the investigation is just a small sample of a large body of data refuting RDA suggestions. Hopefully, the RDA guidelines will soon be adjusted, and suggestions will be based on current scientific data, not speculation.

INVESTIGATION: Richard Harvey and Pamela Champe, the authors of *Lippincott's Illustrated Reviews: Biochemistry*, 3rd ed., said, "The RDA is the average daily dietary intake level that is sufficient to meet the nutrient requirements of nearly all (97–98%) individuals in a life stage and gender group. The RDA is not the minimal requirement for healthy individuals; rather, it is intentionally set to provide a margin of safety for most individuals."

In an article published in 2009 in *Nutrition and Metabolism*, researcher Donald Layman argued that 2010 dietary guidelines should be improved and reflect new understandings about protein requirements. Layman said that according to recent research, "[D]ietary protein intakes above the RDA are beneficial in maintaining muscle function and mobility."

The RDA guideline for protein is 0.8 grams per kilogram of body weight per day. In a study published in 1998 in the *International Journal of Sports Nutrition*, researchers Peter Lemon and colleagues had this to say: "Those involved in strength training might need to consume as much as 1.6 to 1.7 grams per kilogram of bodyweight per day (approximately twice the current RDA) while those undergoing endurance training might need about 1.2 to 1.6 grams per kilogram of bodyweight per day (approximately 1.5 times the current RDA)."

A review by M. Lucas and C. J. Heiss published in 2005 in the *Journal of Aging and Physical Activity* looked at the protein needs of older adults performing resistance training. The researchers concluded that protein intake in older adults that is greater than the RDA increases bone mineral density when calcium intake is adequate; this greater protein intake doesn't appear to compromise kidney health in older individuals with normal kidney function. Individual protein needs for older adults performing resistance training vary according to their health and training regimen, but an intake of 1.0 to 1.3 grams per kilogram of body weight per day should adequately and safely meet their needs, provided that their energy needs are met as well.

Does eating sugar cause obesity?

ANSWER: Sucrose is no different from any other nutrient in its ability to cause weight gain. Is laboratory-made sucrose more likely to cause weight gain than sucrose found in nature? No. Their molecular structures are identical. Eating a moderate amount of sugar is fine, as along as it doesn't lead to overeating or nutritional inadequacies.

INVESTIGATION: When most people talk about sugar, they are referring to sucrose, also called table sugar, which contains one glucose molecule and one fructose molecule. The majority of sucrose consumed in the typical U.S. diet comes from highly processed foods. These foods are often high in calories and low in nutrition. Is sugar the problem or is the problem overconsumption of calorie-dense, nutritionally inadequate foods? The common message is, Don't eat sugar while dieting. Athletes know if they are dieting or preparing for competition that sugar is off-limits; at least, that's what they been told. Is this fear warranted? Is it possible to lose weight while following a diet that contains sugar? Yes, it's possible, as long as you are eating fewer calories than you burn.

Are sweet potatoes more nutritious than white potatoes?

ANSWER: Both potatoes are nutritious, their calorie contents are similar, and they can be eaten with many foods. The assumption that sweet potatoes are more nutritious than white potatoes is often based on the erroneous assumption that white foods are less nutritious than their counterparts.

The following is taken from *Girth Control* (Alan Aragon, 2007):

Sweet Potato Advantages over Russet	Russet Potato Advantages Advantages over Sweet
Higher in fiber (2g more)	Higher in iron and magnesium
Higher in vitamin A	Higher in phosphorus
Higher in B vitamins, except B-6	Higher in potassium
Higher in calcium	Higher in protein
Higher in manganese	Higher in selenium

The belief that sweet potatoes are more nutritious is due to hearsay and misuse of the glycemic index (GI). And, in fact, white potatoes rank high in terms of satisfaction of hunger, higher than any other food ranked.

INVESTIGATION: When I first began bodybuilding, I wouldn't eat white potatoes. My nutritionist advised me to stay away from them. They were bad for my health, he said. And they would make me fat. This notion is usually based on the fact that a white potato ranks higher on the GI (discussed earlier). But a white potato's ranking on the GI doesn't take away its nutritional value. Also, a boiled white potato is the highest-rated food on the satiety index, a tool developed in 1995 by Australian researcher Susanne Holt, PhD, that ranks different foods on their ability to satisfy hunger.

Another consideration when comparing potatoes is the difference in how they are prepared. Sour cream, bacon, cheese, butter, or dressing is often added to white potatoes, significantly increasing the total number of calories. Butter is the only widely popular high-calorie topping for sweet potatoes.

Should I eat the egg yolk?

ANSWER: Yolks are nutritious and the cholesterol content is no big deal for most people. Eating too many yolks may be a bad thing, but too much of *any* food could be bad.

INVESTIGATION: One large egg contains about 5 grams of fat, coming mostly from oleic acid (monounsaturated fat), and 7 to 8 grams of protein. It is loaded with vitamins A and D, riboflavin, folate, and vitamin B-12. The yolk is the most nutrient-dense part of the egg, and is rich in carotenoids, lutein, and zeaxanthin. These carotenoids have positive benefits on the human retina and may decrease age-related vision loss. Why do so many people discard the yolk? Usually, it is fear of its cholesterol content. The media and health officials have exaggerated the dangers of dietary cholesterol. About 70 percent of the population experience little or no increase in cholesterol levels even when their cholesterol intake is high. The body has a feedback loop that inhibits cholesterol production by the body once a certain amount has been ingested.

"We need to acknowledge that diverse healthy populations experience no risk in developing coronary heart disease by increasing their intake of cholesterol, but in contrast, they may have multiple beneficial effects by the inclusion of eggs in their regular diet," said Dr. Maria Luz Fernandez of the University of Connecticut in an article published in 2006 in *Current Opinion in Clinical Nutrition & Metabolic Care*. Dr. Stephen B. Kritchevsky, from Wake Forrest University School of Medicine, discussed the body of epidemiological research on egg consumption in a review published in 2004 in the *Journal of the American College of Nutrition*. In his conclusion, he stated, "In summary, eight studies have reported on the egg consumption and CHD [coronary heart disease] risk directly. On the whole, they do not support the contention that egg consumption is a risk for CHD. However, the largest study is the only one to address the issue specifically. It is also the one that used the best-developed dietary instrument and the most sophisticated analytical approach. This study showed no increase in the risk associated with egg consumption in the general population." A study published in 2005 in the *Journal of Nutrition* by C. M. Greene and colleagues found that the equivalent of three eggs a day for four weeks does not increase the chances of cardiovascular disease in the health of the elderly.

Is the artificial sweetener sucralose unhealthy?

ANSWER: The weight of evidence suggests that sucralose consumption is safe. Splenda is an excellent sugar substitute and contains only 2 calories per teaspoon, versus sugar's 16 calories per teaspoon.

INVESTIGATION: Sucralose is an artificial sweetener discovered in 1976 during a collaborative research program conducted at the Queen Elizabeth College of the University of London. It is made by the selective substitution of sucrose hydroxyl groups with chlorine, resulting in a highly intense, sugarlike sweetness (600 times the sweetness of sugar) and exceptional stability at both high temperatures and low pH. Sucralose is found in the popular sweetener Splenda. Sucralose itself contains no calories. The granular, packet, and tablet forms of Splenda contain a small amount of calories (2 calories per teaspoon) from the bulking agents—maltodextrin, dextrose, and lactose.

In 2000 in *Food Chemical Toxicology*, I. M. Baird reported on two separate studies investigating the tolerance of sucralose by healthy humans. In the first study, sucralose was administered at doses of 1, 2.5, 5, and 10 mg/kg (milligrams of sucralose per kilogram of a person's weight) at 48-hour intervals and followed by daily dosing at 2mg/kg for three days and then 5 mg/kg for four days. In the second study, subjects consumed either sucralose or fructose twice daily in single-blind fashion. Sucralose dosage levels were 125 mg/day for weeks 1 to 3, 250 mg/day during weeks 4 to 7, and 500 mg/day during weeks 8 to 12. No adverse experiences or clinically detectable effects were attributable to sucralose in either study. According to these studies and the extensive animal safety database, there is no indication that adverse effects on human health would occur from frequent or long-term ingestion of sucralose at the maximum anticipated levels of intake. A case study by M. E. Bigal and A. V. Krymchantowski, published in 2006 in *Headache*, found that sucralose consumption contributed to migraines.

Sucralose can be used as a sugar substitute by type 2 diabetics. A study by V. L. Grotz published in 2003 in the *Journal of the American Dietetic Association* investigated the effects of a three-month-long daily administration of high doses of sucralose (7.5 mg/kg/day, or 7.5 mg of sucralose per 1 kg of a person's weight per day) on glycemic control in subjects with type 2 diabetes. The study demonstrated that sucralose consumption at this rate—which is approximately three times the estimated maximum intake—had no effect on glucose homeostasis in individuals with type 2 diabetes. Additionally, the study showed that sucralose was tolerated as well as the placebo.

Do I have to avoid junk food completely to be lean?

ANSWER: The constant availability of tasty junk food has undoubtedly contributed to the country's obesity problem. But other factors, including overindulgence and sedentary lifestyles, must also be considered. Junk food eaten in moderation can go along way toward ensuring dietary success. When people know they will be rewarded—in this case, with junk food—they are more likely to work hard for the reward. With those people who have trigger food issues, the reward system might not work, because it could lead to binge eating.

INVESTIGATION: You probably know someone who seems to always be eating junk food (fries, cakes, chips, and so on) but somehow stays lean. Maybe this person has a high metabolism or some genetic defect? Or maybe eating clean is not required to be lean? Chazz Weaver, author and exercise and nutrition consultant, decided to turn himself into a human guinea pig and answer these questions for himself. His project was featured in a 2005 film *Downsize Me* (a response to Morgan Spurlock's *Super Size Me*). He ate 121 meals from McDonald's in twenty-one days. He exercised, lost 8 pounds, and improved his blood lipid levels. In the summer of 2008, while on a family vacation, I tried the junk food diet and dropped 7 pounds in four days. My activity level was high, which made it possible for me to eat these tasty foods and still drop weight.

Is organic food better for your health than conventional food?

ANSWER: If you like the taste of organic food and have the extra money to spend, go for it. However, don't consider it a necessity. When choosing the foods to include in your diet, the first consideration should be a well-balanced diet. Whether it is made up of conventional or organic foods has little significance.

INVESTIGATION: Over the past two decades, the sale of organic foods has increased nearly 20 percent annually. Today's organic food system includes a combination of small and large food producers, local and global distribution networks, and a wide variety of products, including processed foods, fruits, vegetables, meats, and dairy foods. Recent food crises, such as mad cow disease and foot-and-mouth disease, may have decreased consumer confidence in conventional foods and persuaded them to purchase what they perceive as safer foods—organic foods. In one survey, the reasons people consumed organic foods were to avoid pesticides (70 percent), for freshness (68 percent), for health and nutrition (67 percent), and to avoid genetically modified foods (55 percent). Most organic food advocates I have spoken to eat organic foods because they feel organic foods are safer. "I don't like chemicals in my foods," they say. Or they might say, "Natural has to be safer than artificial." Both statements are erroneous. Organic foods do contain chemicals, and natural is not necessarily safer. Every living molecule inside every living organism is created through chemical reactions. And the natural chemicals contained in organically grown coffee, pepper, mushrooms, apples, celery, potatoes, nutmeg, and carrots present a greater risk of cancer to people than DDT, DDE, or Alar, three pesticides that are banned in the United States and many other countries.

In 2006, the Institute of Food Technologists issued a "Scientific Status Summary" on the organic foods industry. Here is an excerpt from that summary: "Organic fruits and vegetables possess fewer pesticide residues and lower nitrate levels than do conventional fruits and vegetables. In some cases, organic foods may have higher levels of plant secondary metabolites; this may be beneficial with respect to suspected antioxidants such as polyphenolic compounds, but also may be of potential health concern when considering naturally occurring toxins. Some studies have suggested potential increased microbiological hazards from organic produce or animal products due to the prohibition of antimicrobial use, yet other studies have not reached the same conclusion. While many studies demonstrate these qualitative differences between organic and conventional foods, it is premature to conclude that either food system is superior to the other with respect to safety or nutritional composition."

A review published in 2009 in the *American Journal of Clinical Nutrition* investigated the nutritional differences between conventional and organic foods. Eleven crop nutrient categories were analyzed. The researchers identified 162 studies; 55 were of satisfactory quality. Only the satisfactory studies were analyzed. Conventionally produced crops had a significantly higher content of nitrogen, and organically produced crops had a significantly higher content of phosphorus and titratable acidity. There was no difference between the two for the remaining 8 of 11 crop nutrient categories analyzed. Analysis of livestock products indicated no difference in nutrient content between organic and conventional livestock products. After reviewing these studies, the researchers concluded that there was no evidence of a nutritional difference between organic and conventional foods.

Does drinking oxygenated water enhance exercise performance?

ANSWER: In my research, I have found that the consumption of oxygenated water does not enhance aerobic performance and seems to be a marketing gimmick.

INVESTIGATION: Manufacturers of oxygenated water claim that drinking their product produces ergogenic (an increased capacity for mental or physical labor) benefits. A study published in 2006 in the *International Journal of Sports Medicine* investigated the effects of drinking oxygenated water daily for a two-week period. Twenty men with comparable aerobic abilities performed four exhaustive bicycle spiroergometric tests (test measuring maximum oxygen uptake and lung function). Ten subjects drank 1.5 liters of highly oxygenated water every day during the two weeks between the initial two tests. The other ten subjects consumed 1.5 liters of untreated water. After a two-week wash-out period, the subjects underwent a second round of tests while consuming the opposite type of water. Results of the study showed no significant influence on performance parameters. The researchers concluded that drinking oxygenated water did not enhance aerobic performance or kinetics in standardized laboratory testing.

Is a high-fiber diet recommended for everyone?

ANSWER: In general, a moderate- to high-fiber diet offers various health benefits. On the other hand, the importance of fiber is often overemphasized, and much of the supposed health benefits are extrapolated from research on unhealthy individuals and epidemiological studies. Very high-fiber diets may lead to malabsorption of other nutrients. Physique athletes (bodybuilders) often report an improved appearance after discontinuing a high-fiber diet.

INVESTIGATION: In 1972, Hubert Trowell, MD, described dietary fiber as "that portion of food which is derived from cellular walls of plants which is digested very poorly by human beings." Today, the term *dietary fiber* is commonly defined as plant material that resists digestion by the secreted enzymes of the human alimentary tract but which may be fermented by microflora in the colon. In general, a fair amount of dietary fiber should be included in the diet. Some nutritionists suggest up to 40 grams per day. This may be a little much for most people—and way too much for some.

Some health conditions require a low-fiber diet. By reducing the frequency of bowel movements and preventing the irritation of the gastrointestinal tract, a low-fiber diet can be very beneficial for people with diarrhea or abdominal cramping or those experiencing acute phases of ulcerative colitis, regional enteritis, or diverticulitis. A low-fiber diet may also be used postoperatively following a hemorrhoidectomy or large bowel surgery to minimize residue and fecal volume as the patient gradually returns to a regular diet. People experiencing rectal bleeding, partial intestinal obstruction, or constriction of the esophageal or intestinal passageways may also benefit from a low-fiber diet for short periods of time.

Is consuming soy good for your health?

ANSWER: The consumption of soy may benefit your blood lipid profile. But it may also increase your risk of cancer because of the phytoestrogens—which are found in soy—which bind to estrogen

Should I Eat the Yolk?

receptors. Consume soy in moderation and don't rely on it as your primary source of protein.

INVESTIGATION: A meta-analysis published in 2007 in the *American Journal of Clinical Nutrition* investigated the precise effects of soy isoflavones (a group of organic compounds related to flavonoids that act as phytoestrogens in mammals) on lipid (fat) profiles. The researchers found that soy isoflavones significantly reduced serum (the watery fluid of blood) cholesterol and LDL (bad cholesterol) cholesterol but did not change HDL (good cholesterol) cholesterol and triacylglycerol (fat containing glycerol and three individual fatty acids). Soy protein that contained enriched or depleted isoflavones also significantly improved lipid profiles. Reductions in LDL cholesterol were greater in subjects with high levels of cholesterol than in subjects with normal levels of cholesterol.

A meta-analysis published in 2005 in the *American Journal of Clinical Nutrition* looked at the effects of soy protein containing isoflavones on the lipid profile. Soy protein containing isoflavones was associated with significant decreases in serum total cholesterol, LDL cholesterol, and triacylglycerols, and with significant increases in serum HDL cholesterol.

An American Heart Association science advisory has this to say about soy: "[N]o benefit is evident on HDL cholesterol, triglycerides, lipoprotein (a), or blood pressure. Thus, the direct cardiovascular health benefit of soy protein or isoflavone supplements is minimal at best. Soy protein or isoflavones have not been shown to improve vasomotor symptoms of menopause, and results are mixed with regard to the slowing of postmenopausal bone loss. The efficacy and safety of soy isoflavones for preventing or treating cancer of the breast, endometrium, and prostate are not established; evidence from clinical trials is meager and cautionary with regard to a possible adverse effect. For this reason, use of isoflavone supplements in food or pills is not recommended."

44

Are dietary carbohydrates more beneficial than protein for endurance athletes?

ANSWER: Endurance athletes should not neglect eating protein, but they shouldn't neglect carbohydrates either. They are both important for endurance performance. In general, endurance athletes are aware of the need for carbohydrates, but they may not realize the importance of protein. Without sufficient protein, physical development and performance will suffer. In addition to performing better, a sufficient protein intake will help athletes to feel and look better.

INVESTIGATION: The majority of endurance athletes I work with overemphasize their carbohydrate needs and underemphasize their protein needs. To maximize training-induced adaptations, endurance training requires a sufficient amount of protein. A study published in 1998 in the *International Journal of Sports Nutrition* suggests that endurance athletes consume 1.2–1.6 g/kg/day (1.2–1.6 g of protein per 1 kg of a person's weight per day). Another study, this one published in 1988 in the *Journal of Applied Physiology*, found that endurance athletes required 1.67 times more daily protein than sedentary controls. The researchers concluded that endurance athletes required daily protein intakes greater than either bodybuilders or sedentary individuals to compensate for protein breakdown during exercise.

Do sugar alcohols have an effect on blood sugar?

ANSWER: One of the most commonly used sugar alcohols, maltitol and its syrups, does have a significant effect on blood glucose. However, erythritol and mannitol, two sugar alcohols, have no effect.

Four others—lactitol, sorbitol, xylitol, and isomalt—have minimal effect. Different sugar alcohols have different effects on blood glucose.

INVESTIGATION: According to medical writer David Mendosa, several manufacturers of low-carbohydrate products, including Atkins Nutritionals, Biochem, and Keto, say that sugar alcohols have "a negligible effect on blood glucose" or "a minimal impact on blood sugar." Atkins' stance on sugar alcohols is a relatively new development. His 1999 edition of *Dr. Atkins' New Diet Revolution* says, "Sweeteners such as sorbitol, mannitol, and other hexitols (sugar alcohols) are not allowed." Then in 2002, Dr. Atkins published the revised edition of this bestseller, which says that you don't count "non-blood sugar impacting carbs when doing Atkins." These carbohydrates include polydextrose, glycerine, sugar alcohol, and fiber. The Atkins Nutritional Web site says, "We do use fiber and other carbohydrates, such as sugar alcohols, that have a minimal impact on blood sugar and thus fit the Atkins definition of a 'non-digestible' or net carb." (http://atkins.com/Archive/2001/12/21-627515.html; link is no longer available).

A study published in 2003 in *Nutrition Research Reviews* examined the effects of sugar alcohols on the glycemic index (GI). Only two alcohols, mannitol and erythritol, have no impact. Several others have a very low GI, but two maltitol syrups have a GI greater than 50. These are maltitol syrup intermediate and maltitol syrup regular. This is a higher GI value than that of carrots, spaghetti, or orange juice. Dr. Richard K. Bernstein, a noted endocrinologist who authored *Dr. Bernstein's Diabetes Solution*, says that sugar alcohols such as sorbitol will raise blood sugar more slowly than glucose, but still too much and too rapidly to prevent a postmeal blood sugar rise in people with diabetes.

Does carbohydrate loading enhance athletic performance?

ANSWER: I haven't seen any significant benefits with carbohydrate loading. In fact, a few times I felt worse and my performance decreased while carbohydrate loading. My athletes haven't fared any better. In my opinion, the purported benefits of carbohydrate loading are highly questionable. In addition, scientific research does not conclusively support the claim that carbohydrate loading increases athletic performance.

INVESTIGATION: Carbohydrate loading is a technique used to increase the storage of carbohydrate in muscle to levels beyond normal; this is called supercompensation. The procedure requires a carbohydrate depletion phase (a phase in which minimal to no carbohydrates are eaten for at least two to three days in conjunction with a high volume of work), followed by a carbohydrate load phase (a phase in which higher than normal amounts of carbohydrates are eaten for 36 to 72 hours).

Following glycogen (stored glucose) depletion, normal glycogen (stored glucose) levels can be reached in 24 hours. With 36 hours of carbohydrate loading, roughly 150 percent supercompensation can occur. Generally, three to four days of high carbohydrate intake is required to achieve greater levels of muscle glycogen. However, a study published in 2002 in the *European Journal of Applied Physiology* found that combining physical inactivity with a high intake of carbohydrates enables trained athletes to attain maximal muscle glycogen content within only 24 hours. Another study published in 2002 in *Medicine and Science in Sports and Exercise* found that a combination of a short-term bout of high-intensity exercise followed by a high carbohydrate intake enables athletes to attain supranormal muscle glycogen levels within only 24 hours. These studies indicate that the depletion phase isn't necessary for supercompensation to take place. However, many other studies indicate that the depletion process is a key element when attempting to maximize glycogen levels. Supercompensation can be achieved with the correct protocol. But does this increase in carbohydrate storage enhance athletic performance?

In 2003, the *Journal of Applied Physiology* investigated the effects of carbohydrate loading on endurance performance. Eight endurance-trained women were tested. The findings of the study showed that endurance performance was not significantly affected by carbohydrate loading. A study published in 2000 in the *Journal of Applied Physiology* investigated the effects of carbohydrate loading on cycling performance. The study was designed to emulate the demands of competitive road racing. Seven well-trained cyclists performed two 100-km time trials (TTs) on separate occasions, three days after beginning either a carbohydrate-loading or placebo-controlled moderate-carbohydrate diet. The researchers found no difference in performance times or mean power during the TTs.

Do excess carbohydrates in the diet turn into excess body fat?

ANSWER: Normally, de novo lipogenesis (DNL) is not a big player in the formation of body fat. Studies suggest that very high carbohydrate intake or metabolic abnormalities could increase DNL. But significant weight gains via DNL are rare, especially in active individuals.

INVESTIGATION: De novo lipogenesis (DNL) is the metabolic route by which mammals convert excess dietary carbohydrates into fat. Some nutritionists claim that DNL plays a significant role in the development of obesity. Others disagree, saying that DNL's role in the development of obesity is insignificant.

A study published in 1999 in the *European Journal of Clinical Nutrition* pointed out that DNL is not the pathway of first resort for added dietary carbohydrate. In addition, replacement of dietary fat by carbohydrate, when equal in calories, does not induce DNL to a significant degree. The researcher in the study concluded, "DNL is not the pathway of first resort for added dietary CHO [carbohydrate] in humans. Under most dietary conditions, the two major macronutrient energy sources (CHO and fat) are not interconvertible." In 2001 the *American Journal of Clinical Nutrition* examined DNL in lean and obese women in response to both a maintenance calorie diet and a positive calorie diet (a diet with excess calories). The researchers found a significant difference in DNL between the groups when following the maintenance calorie diet, but not when following the positive calorie diet. Although the rates of DNL in the maintenance calorie diet were significantly greater in obese women, the absolute quantities of fat synthesized from carbohydrates during both phases of the diet were relatively small. This study indicates that even when a subject is following a very high-calorie (50 percent over maintenance level), high-carbohydrate diet, the contribution of DNL to body fat is small.

Does calcium intake enhance weight loss?

ANSWER: Most scientific research fails to show that dairy or calcium has any direct, significant effect on weight loss. The effect that calcium or dairy products have on weight loss is secondary to calorie restriction.

INVESTIGATION: Some TV commercials featuring dairy products tell viewers why they should consume dairy: stronger bones, stronger muscles, and increased weight loss. Stronger bones and stronger muscles—sure! Increased weight loss—no.

In a study published in 2004 in the *Journal of Clinical Endocrinology and Metabolism*, researchers examined data from three separate 25-week, placebo-controlled trials to determine whether calcium supplementation during weight loss affects body fat or weight loss. The subjects—100 premenopausal and postmenopausal women—supplemented with 1,000 mg of calcium per day. The researchers found no significant differences in body weight or fat mass between the placebo group and the calcium-supplemented group.

In a study published in 2006 in the *American Journal of Clinical Nutrition*, researchers examined whether calcium supplementation affects body weight and body fat in young girls and whether a relationship exists between habitual calcium intake and body weight and body fat. They found that habitual dietary calcium intake over one year was inversely associated with body fat, but a low-dose calcium supplement had no effect on body weight or body fat in young girls. The researchers suggested that it is possible that the effect of calcium on body weight is exerted only if the calcium is taken as part of a meal. Or, they theorized, the effect might be due to other ingredients in dairy products, and calcium might simply be a marker for a high dairy intake. In a study published in 2005 in the *American Journal of Clinical Nutrition*, researchers investigated the

49

effects of long-term increases in consumption of dairy calcium on body weight and fat mass in young, healthy women. The findings of the study indicated that increased intake of dairy products over one year does not alter body weight or fat mass in young, healthy women.

Do I really need to drink at least 8 glasses of water a day?

ANSWER: Large intakes of fluid, at least "8 X 8" (eight 8-ounce glasses), are advisable for the treatment or prevention of some diseases, such as kidney stones, as well as under special circumstances, such as strenuous physical activity or hot weather. However, most people are currently drinking enough water and, in some cases, more than enough. There is potential harm in drinking too much water. Water intoxication can occur when the kidneys are unable to excrete enough water (as urine). Such instances are not unheard of, and they have led to mental confusion and even death in athletes and nonathletes.

INVESTIGATION: It's common knowledge that we should drink at least eight glasses of water a day. Or is it? Heinz Valtin, a Dartmouth Medical School physician, disagrees. In an invited review published by the *American Journal of Physiology*, Valtin reported that there is no supporting evidence to back up this popular counsel of 8 X 8. How did the 8 X 8 myth start? Valtin thinks that the notion may have started in 1945 when the Food and Nutrition Board of the National Research Council recommended approximately "1 milliliter of water for each calorie of food," which would amount to roughly 2 to 2.5 quarts per day (64 to 80 ounces). In its next sentence the board stated, "[M]ost of this quantity is contained in prepared foods." But that last sentence seems to have been missed, so that the recommendation was erroneously interpreted as how much water a person should drink each day.

Caffeinated beverages and other drinks should also be counted toward daily water intake. University of Nebraska researcher Ann Grandjean published a study in the *Journal of the American College of Nutrition* about the effects of caffeinated beverages on hydration. Grandjean and her colleagues used 18 healthy male adults for their subjects. On four separate occasions, the subjects consumed water or water plus varying combinations of beverages. The beverages were carbonated, caffeinated, caloric, and noncaloric colas and coffee. Body weight, urine, and blood evaluations were performed before and after each treatment. Grandjean found that there were no changes in the body weight, urine, or blood evaluations for the different beverages. The study found no significant differences in the effect of various combinations of beverages on the hydration status of healthy adult males. Therefore, Grandjean concluded that advising people to disregard caffeinated beverages as part of their daily fluid intake is not supported by the results of her study. She went on to say, "[T]he purpose of the study was to find out if caffeine was dehydrating in healthy people who are drinking normal amounts. It is not."

Should athletes drink as much water as they can tolerate?

ANSWER: Good news for athletes: you don't need to carry around a jug of water everywhere you go! Forcing yourself to drink water is not beneficial. Instead, drink when you are thirsty.

INVESTIGATION: In 1996, the drinking guidelines of the American College of Sports Medicine (ACSM) proposed that athletes should drink "as much as tolerable" during exercise. Indeed, many athletes report drinking 1 to 2 gallons of water a day. When I was in my early twenties, I drank at least 1 gallon of water a day. Famous athletes were doing it, and popular fitness magazines reported that drinking large amounts of water was necessary to shed body fat and get fit. Many media sources still advise athletes and exercise enthusiasts to drink as much as they can tolerate. Is there any evidence to support these claims?

In a paper published in the *Journal of Sports Sciences*, Professor Tim Noakes argued that the guideline for athletes to drink as much as they can tolerate during exercise is not supported by evidence. Noakes commented, "If novel universal guidelines for fluid ingestion during exercise are to be promulgated by important international bodies, including the IOC [International Olympic Committee], they should first be properly evaluated in appropriately controlled, randomized, prospective clinical trials conducted under environmental and other conditions that match those found in 'out-of-doors' exercise. This, and the potential influence of commercial interests on scientific independence and objectivity, are the two most important lessons to be learned from the premature adoption of those 1996 ACSM drinking guidelines that are not evidence based."

In a 2006 interview conducted by Louise M. Burke, Noakes explained his findings on fluid intake during sport and exercise. Here is what he had to say: "I reviewed all the published studies in which exercise performance was measured in well-controlled trials in which athletes drank either according to their thirst ('ad libitum') or according to a drinking schedule that insured they drank more, usually 'to replace all the fluid lost as sweat during exercise.' Some studies also included a trial in which athletes drank less than 'ad libitum.' The conclusions were absolutely clear—when athletes drank less than 'ad libitum' they were likely to underperform compared to 'ad libitum' drinking. But there was no study in which drinking more than 'ad libitum' improved performance more than the 'ad libitum' condition. Thus, if we are to be entirely evidence-based in the advice we give athletes, at this moment, we have to say that drinking 'ad libitum' produces the optimum performance."

In other words, drink when you're thirsty.

Can I eat late in the evening if I am trying to lose weight?

ANSWER: Every diet I have ever designed includes a late evening meal; many times it is the biggest meal of the day. If the late evening meal stays within the calorie budget, it will not affect weight loss.

Formulas designed for determining daily calorie maintenance levels are based on calorie expenditure while resting (resting energy expenditure), calorie expenditure required for digestion (thermic effect of feeding), and calorie expenditure due to activity (thermic effect of activity). What time of the day you eat has minimal impact on caloric expenditure.

INVESTIGATION: This myth about restricting food late in the day—which was popular when I was a child—is resurfacing. Some consider eating late as eating past 6 p.m.; others use 7 p.m. or 8 p.m. as their marker. Regardless of their definition of *late*, proponents of this claim generally give the same reasons for not eating in the evening: you are likely to be less active at night and insulin sensitivity is lowest at night. Neither of these reasons is sufficient to support the claim. Many people train late in the evening; post-training, insulin sensitivity is increased. John Ivy, PhD, and Robert Portman, PhD, say that "Immediately after exercise, muscle cells are extremely sensitive to the anabolic effects of the hormone insulin."

Is weight loss slowed by not eating enough?

ANSWER: Skipping a meal here and there or even not eating for a day won't wreck your metabolism. There is no one who won't drop weight if he or she stops eating. I'm not suggesting that dieters stop eating, as long-term starvation can lead to nutrient imbalances and negative health consequences. Generally, moderate calorie reduction is the best way to ensure adherence to a diet and long-term success with it.

INVESTIGATION: An advice columnist in a popular fitness magazine recently stated that the biggest obstacle to people's weight loss efforts was not eating enough. She went on to explain that undereating would slow metabolism and decrease weight loss. Many people accept this statement as fact. However, this idea has been taken out of context and is often misunderstood. In reality, the fastest way you will ever drop weight is to stop eating. With any diet plan, you can expect a drop in resting energy expenditure (REE) after a prolonged period of time. The drop is generally insignificant, doesn't outweigh the decrease in calorie intake, and actually doesn't occur as fast as you might think.

A study published in 1998 in the *American Journal of Clinical Nutrition* investigated the physiological changes that occur during 21 days of starvation in five obese subjects. After three days of starvation, the REE of the subjects actually increased. On day 18, the REE decreased a whopping 8 percent—hardly enough to wreck the metabolism.

Does alcohol consumption cause fat gain?

ANSWER: There are obese people and there are thin people who drink on a regular basis. Obese people who drink also consume too much food. If you are dieting and want to have a drink, that's fine, as long as it's factored into the calorie budget. At the same time, beware of the numerous health and social consequences of too much alcohol.

INVESTIGATION: A person with a potbelly who drinks alcohol on a regular basis is said to have a beer gut. But does drinking alcohol really cause a "beer gut"?

A study published in 1994 in the *American Journal of Clinical Nutrition* investigated the effects of alcohol on post-meal fat storage. The researchers concluded that alcohol has a fat-sparing effect, similar to that of carbohydrates, and will cause fat gain only when consumed in excess of maintenance calorie needs.

Are antioxidants good for my health?

ANSWER: Antioxidants in moderation are good for your health. If you're following a balanced diet that includes fruits, vegetables, whole grains, nuts, and seeds, your antioxidant levels are probably fine. If your diet is lacking in antioxidants, take an antioxidant supplement. Just don't go overboard with supplementation; unnaturally high doses can be harmful to your health. Oxidation is a natural chemical process that occurs in the body and is required for life.

INVESTIGATION: An antioxidant is any molecule that slows down or prevents oxidation reactions. Originally, oxidation reactions were defined as chemical reactions with oxygen, or changes occurring when a substance becomes oxidized (more positively charged). More recently, oxidation reactions have been described as reactions where an atom or molecule loses an electron. Oxidation is a natural part of life. It is excessively high or low antioxidant levels that are detrimental to health.

Some suggest that oxidation reactions contribute to heart disease, declines in cognitive health, and cancer. Vitamin C, vitamin E, and beta-carotene have been shown to act as antioxidants in a test tube; however, this does not mean that they will act as antioxidants in the body. Gerda Endemann, biochemist and author of *Fat Is Not the Enemy*, has this to say: "[E]ven if they [vitamin C, vitamin E, and beta-carotene] act as antioxidants in the body, it is not clear that they will have any effect on heart disease or cancer."

In a five-year study, male smokers with angina (chest pain due to heart disease) were given vitamin E, beta-carotene, both, or a placebo. There was no benefit from any treatment in terms of severe angina or heart attacks. Beta-carotene and vitamin E were actually associated with increased death from heart disease. Male smokers who had previously suffered a heart attack and were taking beta-carotene in this study were 1.75 times as likely to die as were those taking a placebo.

In a study of 18,314 smokers, former smokers, and asbestos-exposed workers published in 1996 in the *New England Journal of Medicine*, the combination of beta-carotene and vitamin A was shown to be possibly harmful, rather than protective. The researchers concluded that "the combination of beta-carotene and vitamin A had no benefit and may have had an adverse effect on the incidence of lung cancer and on the risk of death from lung cancer, cardiovascular disease, and any cause in smokers and workers exposed to asbestos." In another study, beta-carotene (50 mg) or a placebo was given to 22,000 physicians on alternate days for an average of 12 years. There was no difference between the groups in the incidence of heart attacks or deaths from cardiovascular disease.

Another study found that vitamin E was probably effective in reducing the chances of restenosis, the rapid narrowing and hardening of the arteries that can occur immediately following a surgical procedure carried out to open up clogged arteries. In a study published in 2006 in the *Archives of Internal Medicine*, researchers concluded that the long-term use of vitamin E supplements did not provide cognitive benefits among generally healthy older women. A study published in 2003 in the *American Journal of Clinical Nutrition* investigated the effect of high-dose antioxidant supplements on cognition. Information on the use of specific supplements containing vitamins E and C was collected biannually via mailed questionnaires beginning in 1980 from 14,968 community-dwelling women who were registered nurses and participated in the Nurses' Health Study. After looking at the data, the researchers concluded that the use of specific vitamin E supplements—but not specific vitamin C supplements—might be related to modest cognitive benefits in older women.

Is homeopathy an effective treatment for health problems?

ANSWER: A few studies discussing the benefits of homeopathy have appeared in major medical journals. But most positive studies have appeared in nonscientific journals, have been subject to bias, or have had a poor research design. The overwhelming majority of data appearing in scientific journals show that homeopathy is an ineffective treatment for any clinical condition.

INVESTIGATION: Samuel Hahnemann, a German physician, developed homeopathy in the late eighteenth century. He developed homeopathy in response to his dissatisfaction with the conventional medicine of his time. Hahnemann suggested two key principles. First, he asserted that "like cures like"; in other words, a substance that produces certain symptoms in a healthy person can be used to cure similar symptoms in a sick person. Second, he claimed that minute doses of a remedy would be effective. Hahnemann diluted the remedies in a process he named potentization. He would take an original natural substance and dilute it numerous times. Between each dilution, he would shake the remedy. Shaking supposedly released the healing energy of the remedy.

A study published in 1991 in the *British Medical Journal* investigated 107 controlled trials on homeopathy. This is the researchers' conclusion: "At the moment the evidence of clinical trials is positive but not sufficient to draw definitive conclusions because most trials are of low methodological quality and because of the unknown role of publication bias. This indicates that there is a legitimate case for further evaluation of homoeopathy, but only by means of well-performed trials."

A study published in 1990 in *Revue d'Epidemiologie et de Sante Publique* investigated 40 randomized trials involving homeopathy. The researchers concluded that the evidence did not show homeopathy to be effective. In 1994 the National Council Against Health Fraud, a U.S.-based organization, advised consumers not to buy homeopathic products or to patronize homeopathic practitioners. In addition, they stated, "Basic scientists are urged to be proactive in opposing the marketing of homeopathic remedies because of conflicts with known physical laws. Those who study homeopathic remedies are warned to beware of deceptive practices in addition to applying sound research methodologies." A study from 2005 in *Lancet* analyzed 110 trials of homeopathy and 110 conventional medicine trials. The researchers concluded that "there was weak evidence for a specific effect of homoeopathic remedies, but strong evidence for specific effects of conventional interventions. This finding is compatible with the notion that the clinical effects of homoeopathy are placebo effects."

Is sodium bad for my health?

ANSWER: Restriction of salt intake is not advised for the general population. To avoid excess intake of salt, eat foods low in salt, eat high-sodium foods in moderation, and add moderate amounts of salt to foods. In some hypertensive people, the restriction of salt causes a decrease in blood pressure. In others, little or no change occurs. And in yet others, blood pressure may actually increase with salt restriction. Hypertensive individuals should seek medical advice with regard to sodium.

INVESTIGATION: Sodium is essential for life and is classified as a dietary inorganic macro-mineral for animals. Sodium is important for nervous system function and water balance. In general, humans eat significantly more sodium than required. For people with salt-sensitive blood pressure, overconsumption may cause health problems. However, underconsumption may lead to sodium deficiency, or hyponatremia. This condition can be fatal.

For many years, high dietary sodium has been implicated as a cause of hypertension (high blood pressure) and organ damage; yet careful analysis has revealed a weak relationship between sodium intake/excretion and blood pressure in the general population. Studies investigating the effects of dietary sodium reduction on blood pressure have shown only a minimal decrease in blood pressure and no effect on death or cardiovascular health. Although some people do experience large blood pressure changes in response to salt intake, these people are salt sensitive. These individuals experience an increase in blood pressure and body weight when switched from a low-sodium diet to a high-sodium diet. Salt sensitivity is influenced by a number of factors, including genetics, race/ethnicity, age, body mass, and diet, as well as some diseases, including hypertension, diabetes, and kidney dysfunction.

Is aspartame bad for my health?

ANSWER: The FDA says that aspartame is "one of the most thoroughly tested and studied food additives the agency has ever approved." Furthermore, "the more than 100 toxicological and clinical studies it has reviewed confirm that aspartame is safe for the general population." The bulk of existing scientific evidence indicates that aspartame is safe at current levels of consumption as a nonnutritive sweetener.

INVESTIGATION: Aspartame is an artificial sweetener made up of phenylalanine and aspartic acid. The sweetener is marketed under a few brand names, including Canderel, Equal, and Nutrasweet, and can be found in approximately 6,000 products, including diet beverages, dietary supplements, tabletop sweeteners, teas, and desserts. Upon ingestion, aspartame breaks down into its constituent amino acids (phenylalanine and aspartic acid) and free methanol. Aspartame opponents claim that free methanol and phenylalanine present health risks. They might be surprised to find out that the phenylalanine and methanol released from aspartame is small compared with the amount of these substances found in some other dietary sources. An aspartame-sweetened drink contains 20 mg of methanol, an equivalent serving of fruit juice has 40 mg, and an alcoholic beverage contains 60 to 100 mg. A diet soda contains 100 mg of phenylalanine compared with 300 mg for an egg, 500 mg for a glass of milk, and 900 mg for a large hamburger.

Clinical studies have shown no evidence of toxic effects when aspartame is consumed in dosages of 50 mg/kg/day (or 50 mg of aspartame per 1 kg of a person's weight per day). This is equivalent to a 154-pound person drinking 17 cans of diet soda per day. Here is what the American Council of Science and Health says about aspartame: "Numerous authorities, including the Food and Drug Administration, the Joint Expert Committee on Food Additives of the FAO/WHO, the European Community, and the American Medical Association, have concluded that aspartame is a safe product, except in the rare cases of

59

phenylketonuria." The disease referenced—phenylketonuria—is a rare inherited disease that prevents phenylalanine from being properly metabolized.

Is high-fructose corn syrup bad for my health?

ANSWER: The addition of high-fructose corn syrup to a negative energy diet (a diet with fewer calories than are required for maintenance of your current weight) will not cause weight gain. You don't have to get rid of all the sodas in your pantry. Just make sure to drink them in moderation.

INVESTIGATION: In recent years, sucrose has been replaced in many commercial products by high-fructose corn syrup. Corn syrup itself is primarily glucose, which is only about 70 percent as sweet as sucrose. Fructose, however, is about 2.5 times as sweet as glucose. A commercial process has been developed that uses an isomerase enzyme to convert about half of the glucose in corn syrup into fructose. High-fructose corn syrup is just as sweet as sucrose.

The consumption of sugar-sweetened drinks has been linked with obesity in America. A common explanation is that calorie-containing liquids are less filling than solid foods, which leads to overconsumption of calories. However, numerous studies have shown that sugar-containing liquids, when consumed in place of usual meals, may lead to significant and sustained weight loss.

"The hypothesis that fructose, HFCS [high-fructose corn syrup], and caloric beverages play a unique role in obesity and type 2 diabetes beyond their inherent energy contributions has generated tremendous attention from scientists and the media, but no credible scientific support," says John S. White, PhD, and president of White Technical Research. And according to Science Blog (http://www.scienceblog.com/cms/scientists-say-consumers-confused-about-sugars-21934.html), "The American Medical Association helped put to rest a common misunderstanding about high fructose corn syrup and obesity, stating that 'high fructose syrup does not appear to contribute to obesity more than other caloric sweeteners." Even former critics of high fructose corn syrup dispelled myths and distanced themselves from earlier speculation about the sweetener's link to obesity in a comprehensive scientific review published in the December 2008 *American Journal of Clinical Nutrition.*"

CHAPTER 2

EXERCISE CLAIMS

Is it possible to lose stubborn body fat?

ANSWER: Yes, you can lose stubborn body fat. But the recipe is very precise. And doing sit-ups, or any other exercise that targets a particular muscle group, does not contribute to the loss of stubborn body fat.

INVESTIGATION: As the term indicates, stubborn body fat is the fat that is the hardest to shed. Even when a dieter drops fat rapidly in other areas, he or she may hang onto fat reserves in these particular areas. In women, stubborn fat is generally in the hips and thighs. In men, abdominal fat seems to be the hardest to get rid of. Why is some fat so intractable?

All hormones work through specific receptors, and the catecholamines (adrenaline and noradrenaline, which are fat-mobilizing hormones) are no different. They have their own specific receptors called adrenoreceptors. There are two major classes of adrenoreceptors—alpha and beta. And there are two key alpha-receptors, while there are three or maybe four major beta-receptors (one type of beta-receptor is sometimes not included as major because it's found in brown fat cells, which adult humans contain minimal amounts of). When catecholamines bind to alpha-receptors, they decrease fat breakdown. When they bind to beta-receptors, they promote fat loss. This means that catecholamines can act as either fat-mobilizing signalers or anti-fat-mobilizing signalers.

Stubborn fat areas have more alpha-receptors and fewer beta-receptors. Another reason that stubborn fat is so immovable is inadequate blood flow. A sluggish blood flow makes it harder for your blood to transport out free fatty acids during fat breakdown. In response to a meal, blood flow is increased. At all other times, blood flow to stubborn fat is reduced. One of the key ways to attack stubborn fat is to upregulate beta-receptors and downregulate alpha-receptors. There are a few ways to manipulate the action of these adrenoreceptors: increase blood flow to fat cells through aerobic exercise, control insulin levels with a low-carbohydrate diet, and increase thyroid levels (with 25 to 100 mcg/day of thyroid medication).

To shed stubborn fat, high concentrations of adrenaline hormones are required. High levels of adrenaline/noradrenaline mobilize fat but limit its usage as a fuel in muscle. This is why high-intensity exercise is followed by lower-intensity exercise. The high-intensity exercise frees the fat from fat cells; the lower-intensity exercise promotes fat burning. Here is a sample stubborn-fat-burning protocol:

Perform 10 minutes of high-intensity anaerobic or aerobic exercise (or both types of exercise).

Rest for 5 minutes.

Perform 30 minutes of moderate-intensity aerobic exercise.

Author and nutrition consultant Lyle McDonald suggests that the ingestion of oral yohimbe (which contains yohimbine) assists the body in losing stubborn fat. Yohimbine is a selective competitive alpha2-adrenergic receptor antagonist, and 0.2 mg/kg yohimbine (or 0.2 mg of yohimbine per 1 kg of a person's weight) taken once per day inhibits the anti-fat-mobilizing effects of catecholamines. Here is what McDonald says: "Oral yohimbe can be effective when used over the long term. Don't take it within 3–4 hours of taking ephedrine and start with a half-dose to assess tolerance (some people get really freaky responses from it). If you can find pharmaceutical yohimbe, it's far better than the herbal version.

(Most of the herbal versions are crap...) Taking the yohimbine with caffeine prior to morning cardio does seem to help with very stubborn fat."

Will gaining muscle speed up my metabolism?

ANSWER: Research has found that muscle burns only slightly more calories than fat.

INVESTIGATION: If you have been around the fitness industry very long, or even read any of the popular fitness magazines, you have probably heard that muscle tissue burns way more calories than fat tissue does. So one of the best ways to lose body fat is to add more muscle to your frame, right? This was what I believed—until a recent review of the primary scientific research revealed something surprising.

A paper published in 2001 in *Current Opinion in Clinical Nutrition and Metabolic Care* gives a detailed description of calorie requirements for various organs and tissues while at rest. I had always heard that 1 pound of skeletal muscle, while at rest, burned 40 to 60 calories a day. This statement turned out to be a myth. Scientific data reveals that 1 pound of muscle burns fewer than 6 calories a day, while 1 pound of fat burns approximately 2 calories a day. So if you were to exchange 20 pounds of fat for an equivalent amount of muscle, your metabolic rate would increase so that you burned approximately 80 more calories a day. That's the number of calories in a small to medium piece of fruit!

Will performing sit-ups shrink my waistline?

ANSWER: Sit-ups do not shrink the waistline. To shrink the waistline, you need to drop body fat. Sit-ups should be included in a comprehensive fitness program, but the idea that they somehow decrease the size of the waist is a fairy tale.

INVESTIGATION: Slimming the stomach and trimming the waistline are probably the most discussed topics in the fitness industry. Tummy-shrinking infomercials fill late-night TV slots. And magazines are filled with superab ads. What's the deal? Do sit-ups, in fact, shrink the waistline?

According to Alan Aragon, nutrition researcher and author of *Girth Control*, this is a myth. In addition to exercise, calories need to be burned. "It's not sit-ups per se that shrink the waistline, it's whether or not you're losing body fat by remaining in a net caloric deficit over a period of weeks or months. Training a muscle doesn't automatically disintegrate the fat surrounding it," Aragon said in a recent conversation via e-mail.

Will exercise get rid of cellulite?

ANSWER: Most women can lessen the effects of cellulite with a quality training and nutrition regimen. Note that even some very lean women have cellulite.

INVESTIGATION: Cellulite is the dimpling of skin caused by the protrusion of subcutaneous fat into the skin. Between 85 and 98 percent of adult women display some degree of cellulite. It is prevalent in women of all races, but is even more common in Caucasians than in Asians. There appears to be a hormonal component to cellulite. It is rarely seen in men.

These factors are important to a cellulite-reduction regimen: losing fat, dropping extracellular fluid, inducing muscular growth, and strengthening connective tissue. Some women significantly decrease cellulite by following a quality exercise and nutrition regimen. Others drop a great deal of weight but only minimally reduce the appearance of cellulite. Some women use creams and some choose surgery. Some studies show that some creams have promising results while other studies show no effects from the same formula. The best plan is to use a cream in combination with exercise and nutrition. Surgery should be your *last* choice. Before you decide to have surgery, consider the fact that cellulite poses no health risk, but surgery always poses a health risk.

Will my muscle turn to fat if I stop weight training?

ANSWER: Muscle does not turn to fat. If you stop working out, you will probably lose a fair amount of muscle and possibly gain a fair amount of fat.

INVESTIGATION: Muscle and fat are different types of tissue. They are not interconvertible. If you stop training, you no longer have the appropriate stimuli to promote muscle gains. If you continue to eat the same as you did when training, your caloric intake will surpass your daily maintenance calorie requirement—resulting in fat gain. Even under these conditions, some of the calories will be allocated to muscle. Genetics plays a large role in how much weight gain contributes to fat tissue and how much it contributes to muscle tissue.

If I train hard enough, will I look like a pro bodybuilder?

ANSWER: Few individuals will ever look like a pro bodybuilder. I say that not to be discouraging, but to be factual. Becoming a pro bodybuilder requires painstaking, hard work, proper genetics, and sacrifice. Even most people with the right genetics are not willing to go to the lengths required to attain pro bodybuilder status.

INVESTIGATION: If a person has the right genetics, works hard, and has access to performance-enhancing drugs, then he or she could become a pro bodybuilder.

First, let's talk about genetics. Pro bodybuilders have genetics that allow them to gain unusual levels of muscle tissue. Their ability to synthesize muscle proteins is very high, and the time availability for synthesizing these proteins is prolonged. Some studies indicate that pro bodybuilders have a mutated myostatin gene, a gene that regulates muscular growth.

Now, let's discuss hard work. This includes weight training on a regular basis and adherence to a strict diet. The diet is the hardest part for most bodybuilders. Most people cringe when they see the precise, rigorous diets that bodybuilders follow.

Last, but not least, let's talk about performance-enhancing drugs. These drugs are a key element in the pro bodybuilder regimen—at least for those bodybuilders competing in non-natural shows. "Natural" bodybuilding shows are drug tested; shows that are not designated as natural are not drug tested.

The most common performance-enhancing drugs are anabolic-androgenic steroids (AAS). These drugs are illegal, pose health risks, and are expensive. Pro bodybuilders have access to a large array of these drugs, which act to increase muscle protein synthesis and decrease protein breakdown. AAS users have a big advantage over naturals when it comes to gaining and preserving muscle.

Are hanging leg raises a good exercise for the abdominals?

ANSWER: Hanging leg raises are a great exercise for the hip flexors—but they have little dynamic effect on the abdominals. The abdominals plays a stabilizing role in this movement, but not a dynamic role, as many sources claim. You can increase the dynamic activity of the abdominals by crunching the torso and performing a pike movement while raising the legs.

INVESTIGATION: Hanging leg raises are a popular exercise in commercial gyms. Fitness magazines often recommend this movement as part of the abdominal routine. I like this movement and incorporate it into my own training regimen. But the abdominal muscles play a stabilizing role in this movement, not the dynamic role that many sources claim. The abdominals prevent any significant movement of the pelvis, while the primary muscle group involved in this exercise is actually the hip flexors. If you crunch the torso, performing a pike movement while raising the legs, the dynamic activity of the abdominals increases.

Is weight training safe for children?

ANSWER: A properly designed weight-training program can be beneficial for growing children. Weight training is less likely to have a negative impact on growth than many other sports.

INVESTIGATION: Weight training for children has been taboo in the United States for decades. I am sure that you have heard it said that weight training is unsafe for children. Some have even commented that weight training is bad for the joints and stunts growth. Yet there is no evidence to support these claims. In reality, the risks appear to be far less with weight training than with football, running, basketball, and other popular sports. Biomechanical research has shown that activities such as throwing, running, and hitting impose larger forces on the body than weight training. These activities have been shown to place heavier stress on the growth plates of growing bones than weight training does.

Studies show that children who weight train have higher bone mineral densities, which indicates benefits to bone strength. Eastern European countries have found that children are significantly healthier when they engage in proper weight training. The American Society of Pediatrics and the American Orthopedic Society for Sports Medicine have said that weight training can be positive for children. These organizations have stated the need for careful workout planning, proper biomechanics, and supervision by a qualified trainer.

Consider the following when designing a weight-training program for children: rarely attempt one repetition maximums (only when properly supervised, after learning proper technique, and when not fatigued); emphasize proper technique; set realistic goals; supervise young athletes; and provide individualized programs for young athletes.

Are seated exercises safer than standing ones?

ANSWER: It is important to be aware of back positioning and to have a strong enough core when performing either seated or standing exercises. Proper positioning means that the chest is up, the shoulders are back, and the lower back is held in a tight arch. Even when concentrating on holding this position, some people fail; this usually implies a weak core. Seated exercises are no safer than standing exercises and, in fact, may actually be more dangerous.

INVESTIGATION: The claim that seated exercises are safer than standing exercises is often perpetuated by the fitness media and gym owners, who promote the use of "machines only" when weight training. They claim that seated exercises prevent stress in the lower back, and that performing standing exercises increases the risk of back injury. What does the research say? According to Mel Siff, PhD, and author of *Facts and Fallacies of Fitness*, research reveals that erect, relaxed, and unloaded sitting alone can increase stress on the lumbar spine by 40 percent. And if the back is rounded while sitting, lumbar loading can almost double.

Will wearing a lifting belt weaken my midsection?

ANSWER: The appropriate use of a lifting belt *increases* abdominal strength. Wearing a belt when lifting heavy weights is strongly suggested. To use a belt properly, adjust the belt so that it is tight, push the abdominals out against the belt, and hold your breath. A belt, properly used, becomes increasingly important as the weights get heavier.

69

INVESTIGATION: Some trainers and coaches claim that wearing a belt, which increases intra-abdominal pressure, weakens the abdominal muscles. It is presumed that this imposes excessive stress on the lumbar disks, thus promoting their degeneration.

According to Mel Siff, author of *Facts and Fallacies of Fitness*, using a belt can help to increase, rather than decrease, abdominal strength. External pressure exerted on the abdominals when using a belt correctly increases tension, thus strengthening the midsection.

Are knee extensions more effective than squats for knee rehabilitation?

ANSWER: Knee extensions cause more stress on the knee than squats do. Generally, a multijoint movement, such as squats, is the better choice when addressing knee rehabilitation. Start with a light weight, and increase the weight slowly. Practice controlled movement and good technique.

INVESTIGATION: Research indicates that patella femoral and soft tissue forces are greater during knee extensions than during well-controlled squats. In other words, there is more force on the knee during knee extensions than during squats. Seated knee extensions prevent the hip joint from sharing the loading of the movement. In addition, the controlled line of movement doesn't offer the natural patterns of linked joint movement, nor does it involve the central nervous system in producing natural daily patterns of motor control. Remember that there are different types of squats, and that the speed of movement varies. The popular claim that you shouldn't do squats fails to recognize these factors. Different types of squats provide the body with different stresses. Finally, consider the type of knee injury. Certain types of squats are more conducive to rehabilitation of certain types of knee injuries than others are.

Is low-intensity, long-duration aerobics the best exercise for fat loss?

ANSWER: Contrary to hearsay, you do not have to do low-intensity, long-duration aerobics to lose fat. Keep in mind when considering net fat loss that the fat burned while training is only part of the picture. Post workout, 24-hour, and long-term fat loss must be considered. Both high-intensity and low-intensity exercise can help to attain fat loss. When pressed for time, high-intensity, short-duration exercise may be the practical choice; at other times, you may prefer low-intensity, long-duration exercise.

INVESTIGATION: Dietary factors excluded, the proportional burning of fat during exercise is related to training intensity. The lower the intensity, the greater the proportion of stored fat burned; the higher the intensity, the less the proportion of fat burned.

Remember, a higher proportion does not necessarily indicate a higher total. Consider this scenario. Subject A burns 10 units of energy and 80 percent of those units are fat, while subject B burns 15 units of energy and 70 percent of those units are fat. In this scenario, subject A burned 8 units of fat while subject B, who burned a smaller proportion of fat, burned 10.5 units of fat. So the real question is what type of exercise causes net fat loss? When addressing this question, consider that the actual time spent training takes up a small portion of an entire day. Even if you train two hours a day, there are still twenty-two hours when you are not training. It may surprise you to learn that, as you're sitting there reading this, you are burning proportionally more fat than you would be sprinting 100 meters. But sprinting 100 meters would be more beneficial than reading for fat loss. Which one of these activities burns more calories?

A study published in 2002 in the *Journal of Applied Physiology* compared healthy men and women, ages 20 to 45, who burned the same amount of calories exercising at 40 percent VO2 max (maximum oxygen uptake in liters per minute) or 70 percent VO2 max. There was no difference in net fat oxidation between the low-intensity and high-intensity groups at the 24-hour mark. A study published in 2004 in the *International Journal of Obesity and Related Metabolic Disorders* looked at obese males using a high-intensity, interval protocol versus a low-intensity, linear one. There was no difference in fat oxidation between the high-intensity and low-intensity treatments at 24 hours. In addition, the high-intensity group actually burned a higher proportion of fat post exercise. Long-term tests are the most important when looking at total fat loss. A common finding with long-term testing is that when calorie expenditure is the same with high-intensity and low-intensity exercises, minimal differences are seen in fat loss. Another finding generally suggests that high-intensity training results in maintenance or growth of muscle tissue, and low-intensity training results in loss of muscle tissue.

Does wearing strength shoes increase strength?

ANSWER: Research has shown that wearing strength shoes does not increase strength—and may be dangerous.

INVESTIGATION: A study published in 1993 in the *American Journal of Sports Medicine* evaluated the effectiveness and safety of a strength shoe–training regimen designed for increasing strength in intercollegiate track and field participants. No gains in strength were reported in the participants wearing the strength shoes at the end of the eight-week training program. The authors concluded that the strength shoe couldn't be recommended as a safe, effective training method for developing lower leg strength. The results of this study did not surprise me. The mechanical factors involved with wearing strength shoes are not conducive to increases in strength. In most cases, training with a fancy gadget, such as this one, leads to a deconditioned athlete.

Does wearing strength shoes increase flexibility?

ANSWER: Wearing strength shoes does not increase flexibility. And if they are worn for extended periods of time, they might *decrease* ankle flexibility, due to the long duration of plantar flexion (the movement where the top of the foot moves away from the shin).

INVESTIGATION: A study published in 1993 in the *American Journal of Sports Medicine* investigated the effectiveness of the strength shoe-training regimen for increasing flexibility. No benefits for flexibility were found.

To gain muscle, must I do 3 sets of 10 repetitions of each exercise?

ANSWER: When working to gain muscle, the weights you use should get progressively heavier, and the total work (weight multiplied by total number of repetitions) should increase. There is no magic set-repetition scheme. The "3 X 10" myth was probably based on the DeLorme method. The classic DeLorme method involved 3 sets of 10 repetitions—50 percent of 10RM (10 repetition maximum) for the first set, 75 percent of 10RM for the second set, and 100 percent of 10RM for the last set.

INVESTIGATION: I used to work with a trainer who swore by the 3 X 10 mantra: 3 sets of 10 repetitions if you want to be muscular. I tried to discuss the 3 X 10 rule with the trainer a few times, but he never really wanted to go into depth about his reasoning beyond "That's the way big guys train." In reality, big guys train using a variety of set and repetition schemes. Some prefer more repetitions and lighter weights; others like fewer repetitions using heavier weights.

Dan Moore, founder of Hypertrophy-Research.com, reported on a study that compared a low-volume protocol (3 sets of 2 or 3 repetitions of squats) with a high-volume protocol (3 sets of 9 or 10 repetitions of squats) over a six-week period. Both groups increased their thigh size, but there was no significant difference between the groups.

Will high-repetition weight training make me lean?

ANSWER: High-repetition weight training does not make people lean. Furthermore, if done to excess, high-repetition weight training can cause a significant loss of muscle tissue, especially when performed while following a low-calorie diet.

INVESTIGATION: Many individuals who are trying to get lean perform high-repetition weight training. This type of training often appears to cause significant fat loss. But when looking beneath the surface, we find that there is more to weight loss than just training. "Although exercise does increase energy output during and after exercise and can expend energy from fat for many overweight persons, excessive caloric expenditure has limited implications for substantially reducing body weight independent of nutritional modifications," says weight loss researcher C. J. Zelasko. In other words, modify your caloric intake as well as your caloric expenditure.

Is it dangerous to lock the knees while exercising?

ANSWER: Locking the knees is a natural occurrence during movement. Suggesting that you must never lock the knees while exercising is bad advice. Locking the knees decreases the chances of rotational injuries, and locking the knees during exercise can contribute to knee joint strength.

INVESTIGATION: In everyday activities, the knees are locked on a regular basis while standing and lifting. Olympic weightlifters and power lifters lock their knees intensively while lifting ultraheavy loads. Imagine someone following you around all day, telling you not to lock your knees when you stand or when you lift something. Sounds silly, doesn't it? So why isn't it silly when trainers in the gym give essentially the same advice? On another note, these same trainers often fail to mention the possibility of knee injury due to rotation of the knee, which can occur only when the knee is bent. Locking the knee can prevent injuries that occur due to rotation.

Should I avoid back exercises if I have back problems?

ANSWER: Back injury is very painful in some cases. For fear of further pain, many people with back injuries avoid exercise. But this attempt at lessening pain often results in a worsening condition. In most cases, people with lower back problems shouldn't avoid exercise. But they should approach exercise with caution. Special attention should be focused on technique when doing seated back exercises, as these exercises promote increased loading of the lumbar spine and rounding of the lower spine, both of which can negatively affect back health.

INVESTIGATION: Avoidance of back exercises usually causes back problems to worsen. Prone (lying face down) leg raises or prone trunk extensions on the mat are good exercises for people with severe back injuries, but offer little strengthening for those with less-severe injuries. Prone leg raises work the gluteus maximus dynamically but not the erectors (the muscles in the lower back). Prone trunk exercises work the erectors over a small range, which isn't similar to how the back is used in daily life or sports. To strengthen the back, exercises must be performed in a progressive manner, in which load and total work are increased.

Is aerobic exercise recommended for all athletes?

ANSWER: Approximately 80 to 85 percent of sports are classified as anaerobic (without oxygen) activities. Aerobic exercise provides minimal benefits for these athletes, and can actually be detrimental, although long-duration aerobics may provide psychological and recovery benefits. Mental toughness is a benefit sometimes gained from long-duration activities. A certain amount of mental toughness is required to keep going when you're tired and sweaty. Some research and anecdotal evidence suggest that aerobic activity may speed up recovery from exercise, which is beneficial to all athletes. A moderate amount of aerobic activity has its role, but too much is not a good thing.

INVESTIGATION: Excessive aerobic endurance training can have negative effects on protein synthesis, strength, power, speed, agility, and quickness, while moderate aerobic endurance training will neither negatively nor positively affect these qualities. It's not unusual to see baseball players, football players, and volleyball players—athletes who are involved in speed strength sports—performing a great deal of aerobic exercise. Should these athletes spend so much time doing aerobic exercise? They should not.

The following quotes are from the Supertraining Discussion Forum (supertraining@yahoogroups.com [accessed November 19, 2001]), a forum that was founded by the late Mel Siff, PhD, and author of *Supertraining*:

"Endurance training reduces the inherent capability of the neuromuscular system for maximum power output (Dudley & Fleck, 1987)."

"Vertical jumping ability—inherently a fast-twitch muscle function—decreases with endurance training (Bosco et al., 1983; Ono et al., 1976)."

"Endurance training performed concurrently with weight training (e.g., an every other day approach) interferes with optimal strength, power and size development in muscles involved (Hickson, 1980; Dudley & Djamil, 1985)."

"Concurrent endurance training and weight training markedly interferes with an athlete's ability to perform explosive movements, due mainly to adaptive responses in the muscle (Hickson, 1980; Dudley & Djamil, 1985; Dudley & Fleck, 1987)."

Is circuit training the best way to maximize fitness levels?

ANSWER: Circuit training is time efficient, good for beginners, and can be used to increase general physical preparation levels. However, circuit training does not develop optimal levels of fitness.

INVESTIGATION: Circuit training is a hot topic in the fitness industry. Many fitness gurus promote circuit training as the best and fastest way to attain all-around fitness. Contrary to what many circuit-training advocates say, it is not a new training method.

According to the Gym Jones Web site, Morgan and Adamson in England developed circuit training during the 1950s for use with beginning fitness students (as compared with fit athletes) in school physical education classes. The goal of circuit training was to develop the four aspects of general or athletic fitness simultaneously: strength, power, muscular endurance, and circulo-respiratory endurance. Morgan and Adamson stressed that circuit training should focus on individual needs. The majority of circuit training seen in today's gyms is anything but individualized. Everyone performs the same workout.

Scientific research has found that circuit training produces inferior results compared with the cumulative effects of separate training sessions, each devoted to enhancing different types of fitness.

Should I Eat the Yolk?

In *Supertraining*, author Mel Siff says this: "[A]ll forms of circuit training are largely suited to the average non-athlete or competitive athlete during the early preparatory phase of training. The constant progression in a circuit from one exercise to another, without completing all sets with one exercise to a prescribed maximum number of repetitions before moving to the next exercise, does not permit one to adequately develop the different types of sport-specific strength. Even with interval circuit training on machines, it is not possible to train with the medium heavy, near maximal or explosive loading, which is necessary to develop qualities such as muscle hypertrophy (muscular growth), speed-strength, strength-speed, static strength, flexibility-strength, explosive strength, and acceleration strength."

Will heavy weight training make me bulky?

ANSWER: Heavy weight training strengthens muscles, bones, and connective tissue. Even when following a program that incorporates heavy weight training, it is difficult for most people—especially women—to attain high levels of muscularity.

INVESTIGATION: If achieving bulk were easy, there would be a bunch of happy men worldwide. In reality, a proper resistance-training program, in conjunction with sufficient nutrition, enhances muscularity. In order to gain extraordinary amounts of muscle, you need the right genetics, the right nutrition, and the right training environment. "Getting too big" is a fear commonly expressed by female trainees. In many cases, however, extremely muscular women are as big as they are because they supplement with high doses of anabolic-androgenic steroids.

Will heavy weight training make me slow?

ANSWER: Heavy weight training has the potential to enhance your speed significantly. Many successful sprinters incorporate heavy weight training into their programs.

INVESTIGATION: Sprinters are among the fastest—perhaps the fastest—people in the world. Heavy weight training is a key element in the sprinter's conditioning program. Several researchers have shown that speed of movement increases with muscular strength. I have seen many athletes increase their speed simply by getting stronger. This occurs most often in novice athletes. Sprinters, Olympic lifters, and football players, as well as most athletes participating in speed power sports, train with heavy weights.

Does heavy weight training decrease flexibility?

ANSWER: Performing full-range-of-motion strength-training movements, such as squats, side presses, and Olympic lifts, enhances flexibility. In most cases, even if you get muscular, heavy weight training will not decrease your flexibility. Some skinny people lack flexibility, just as some muscular people lack flexibility. Competitive gymnasts and cheerleaders are good examples of athletes who are both very muscular and very flexible.

INVESTIGATION: Olympic lifts are often performed with very heavy weights. When measuring overall flexibility, Olympic weightlifters as a group rank second only to gymnasts. Performing the Olympic lifts requires a high level of flexibility. There is no better exercise than the snatch, an Olympic lift, for flexibility.

79

Do big muscles equal big strength?

ANSWER: A variety of factors contribute to strength. The size of the muscle is one factor among many. And a big muscle is not necessarily a strong muscle.

INVESTIGATION: Strength is determined by more than just structural factors (size of muscle and body mass). I have seen big, muscular guys fail to demonstrate any appreciable amount of strength. To exhibit strength, the nervous system and muscles must work in a coordinated fashion.

Strength is proportional to the cross-section area of muscle. Therefore, larger muscles have the potential to develop greater strength than smaller muscles. However, some Olympic weightlifters, power lifters, and other athletes consistently increase strength while maintaining the same body mass.

Here are some of the key factors that determine strength:

- Cross-sectional area of muscle
- Mechanical leverage across the joint
- Density of muscle fibers per unit of cross-sectional area
- Motor unit recruitment (the simultaneous contraction of numerous muscle fibers)

The book *Supertraining* (Siff, 2000) details lists of factors that contribute to strength. Many factors contribute to strength, and there are various types of strength, including maximum strength, speed strength, and strength endurance. A detailed description of the different types of strength are beyond the scope of this book. However, *Supertraining* is an excellent source for more information about different types of strength training.

A workout designed to increase strength should be based on two key principles: (1) progressive increases in the amount of weight used, and (2) progressive increases in total work. Basically, work equals weight times the total repetitions.

Is light weight training safer than heavy weight training?

ANSWER: Heavy weight training can be dangerous, particularly when performed by novices, children, or unhealthy individuals. However, light weight training can also be dangerous, especially if you perform while fatigued or with improper technique. Practice caution when using heavy or light weights.

INVESTIGATION: According to Newton's second law (The force involved is proportional to the acceleration of the object), light weights can produce greater forces in the muscles than heavy weights if moved fast enough. And more injuries occur in sports and activities that use no added resistance at all (for example, running, soccer, or aerobics) than occur with heavy weight training.

Is projecting the knees over the toes while exercising dangerous to the knees?

ANSWER: There are specific health conditions where it's important to avoid this movement, but in general, this claim does not apply to healthy populations.

INVESTIGATION: In everyday life and sporting activities, there are hundreds of situations where the knee projects over the toe. These activities include wrestling, sprinting, walking up stairs, Olympic weightlifting, and any general sports movement. Why is this movement not permitted during exercise? This advice has been given for so long that some have come to accept it as fact. In reality, this fact is nothing more than fitness industry dogma.

The next time you see someone walking up the stairs, look at his or her knee position. Where is the knee in relation to the toes? Chances are, the knee is projecting over the toes. This is a natural movement pattern that is not considered "bad," unless you are exercising. According to Mel Siff in *Facts and Fallacies of Fitness*, "Many aboriginal folk squat many times a day while carrying out their daily chores, while the Japanese sit on the floor with their knees fully flexed beneath them bearing all their bodyweight for prolonged periods daily without producing an epidemic of knee injuries."

Should I pull in my stomach during exercise?

ANSWER: Pulling in your stomach decreases spinal stabilization and can be dangerous, especially when lifting heavy weights. You want to be strong when lifting weights, so hold your breath and push out your stomach.

INVESTIGATION: Pulling in the stomach during exercise can result in serious injury when weight training. Sucking in the stomach causes spinal flexion and decreases intra-abdominal pressure, which results in decreased spine stabilization. And spinal stabilization is important when exercising, especially when using heavy weights. To increase spine stabilization, hold your breath and expand your midsection.

Are standing dumbbell flies a good exercise for the chest?

ANSWER: To stimulate the chest, lie down when performing dumbbell flies. The standing version of the exercise does little to stimulate the chest, although it is a decent exercise for the shoulders.

INVESTIGATION: The chest muscles are mildly involved when performing standing dumbbell flies. Using heavy dumbbells doesn't make the chest work any harder, but it does make the shoulders work harder, to keep the arms from dropping.

Are "good mornings," a lower back exercise, dangerous?

ANSWER: If performed properly, good mornings are a great developmental tool for the posterior chain (glutes, lower back, and hamstrings). They can also be dangerous under some conditions. Begin with a very light weight when learning this exercise. Be sure that your technique is good before moving on to heavier weights. Do not attempt 1-repetition maximums (the maximum amount of weight you can lift once) with this exercise.

INVESTIGATION: When performing good mornings, most of the forward bending should occur at the hip joint rather than the vertebrae; the lower back should be held tight and arched; and the bar should be held across the upper shoulders, with the knees slightly bent and the buttocks thrust backward. The movement should be performed in a controlled fashion. The potential for injury increases when forward bending involves vertebral flexion rather than hip flexion, spinal flexion with rotation, or an excessive range of motion. The movement also becomes unsafe if your load is too heavy, if your knees are locked, if your glutes aren't pushed backward, or if you perform with uncontrolled speed or until fatigued (this compromises technique).

Are squats better for the glutes than lunges are?

ANSWER: Both of these exercises stimulate the glutes. Keep in mind that there are various types of squats and lunges. All variations are not created equal; some are more difficult and require more athleticism. In addition to developing the glutes, these exercises will benefit the legs, lower back, and hips.

INVESTIGATION: The glutes are extensors of the hips, and any exercise that promotes hip extension, such as squats, deadlifts, waiter's bows, or lunges, will develop these muscles. The degree of hypertrophy (muscular growth) in this area depends on the load used, genetics, total work, and nutritional protocol. If you are doing movements that involve hip extension, you are training the glutes.

Is it safer to use a suspended walking machine than to walk or run?

ANSWER: Suspended walking machines do not provide the safety that sellers claim. In fact, their use can have negative impacts on health. A key selling point for suspended walking machines is "little to no impact." In everyday locomotive activities, the body is subjected to varying degrees of impact. Exercise should prepare the body for impact; exercising on suspended walking machines does not do this.

INVESTIGATION: These are the Sky Walker machines you have probably seen on late-night television. The infomercials say that using them is safer than walking or running, and that the machines minimize impact and are fun. Is using one of these machines really safer than walking or running?

When you use the suspended walking machine, you rely primarily on your hip flexors and extensors but minimize the use of your quadriceps, hamstrings, plantar flexor muscles, and other major walking and running muscles. This abnormal movement pattern can heighten stress on the hips and lumbar area. The lack of involvement of the major walking and running muscles minimizes the overall training effects. The proposed benefit of completely eliminating impact to the body actually results in a serious disadvantage. Impact loading as a result of controlled walking and running offers important benefits to the musculoskeletal system.

This is what Mel Siff, PhD, and author of *Facts and Fallacies of Fitness*, says: "[J]oints subjected to heavy impacts such as the ankle are relatively free from osteoarthritis in old age, and those that are subjected to much lower loading experience a greater incidence of cartilage fibrillation and osteoarthritis." In addition, Siff says, "Healthy cartilage is cartilage that is subjected to repetitive, physiological loading regularly, and this includes full proper joint motion during exercise. Zero impact machines that hold joints immobile while subjecting them to compression and variations on this theme are bound to be very bad for the health of chondrocytes and cartilage metabolism. Soft, irregularly loaded cartilage is cartilage that eventually deteriorates."

Do lying leg press machines, or leg sleds, train the legs without stressing the back?

ANSWER: If your back hurts or is injured, you need to take special measures to reduce spinal loading. Lying leg press machines, or leg sleds, do not relieve stress to the lower back. If you still choose to use these machines, be cautious and use light loads.

INVESTIGATION: Lying leg press machines are commonly used by individuals who want to exercise the legs while eliminating heavy loading from the back. Keep in mind that any form of pressure on the head, shoulders, or feet increases spinal compression and intervertebral loading. Lying down does decrease spinal compression, but as soon as longitudinal loading begins, spinal stress increases. That isn't necessarily a bad thing. Spinal loading is necessary to increase spinal strength.

Do machine exercises provide stress in the same way as their free weight equivalents?

ANSWER: Machines have their role in training, but they do not offer the same benefits as free weight training. Athletes should use machines sparingly.

INVESTIGATION: Machine advocates claim that machine movements mimic the movements of their free weight equivalents but are much safer (for example, seated shoulder press substituted for the free weight equivalent, the standing dumbbell press). Most machines (with the exception of cable devices, which are free to move in three-dimensional paths) force the user to follow two-dimensional, linear paths of motion (in real life, the body can move in a three-dimensional, multiplanar pathway). Use of these machines can result in imbalances in muscular development and reductions in motor proficiency in other activities, especially competitive athletics. Remember, training relies not only on muscular development but also on movement patterns. An overreliance on fixed pathway machines tends to weaken your natural proprioceptive abilities (these abilities develop based on your own body's stimulus and are important to coordination, balance, and posture). Fixed pathway machines also tend to weaken your stabilization and range of motion.

Does being lean mean that I am fit?

ANSWER: Leanness is not the same as fitness. Fit people come in all shapes and sizes. In fact, being *too* lean can even be detrimental to health and sports performance. I experienced the negative effects of being too lean while kickboxing. My skin was bruised and my joints were sore on a regular basis. These problems disappeared once I put on a little weight.

INVESTIGATION: How many times have you heard someone say, "Hey, I saw this really fit guy (or girl) at the mall; I want to look just like that"? When I hear this statement, I ask, "How do you know that person is fit?" It's a mistake to classify someone as fit based on appearance alone. Look at people from various sports and you will see that many types of body shapes are successful. That said, even being good at a particular sport does not mean that you are fit. What constitutes fitness? There is no definitive answer to this question, but according to most research, being fit requires at least a moderate level of various qualities of fitness, including speed, strength, stamina, flexibility, and balance. Many lean individuals are fit, but even more lean individuals are not fit.

Can Pilates exercises lengthen my muscles?

ANSWER: Pilates exercises do not permanently lengthen the muscles. If this were to occur, after a while you would be immobilized. Full-range-of-motion weight training increases flexibility. For example, Olympic weightlifters are among the most flexible people in the world.

INVESTIGATION: Pilates advocates claim that weight training tends to shorten the muscles, but Pilates lengthens them. They also claim that lifting weights makes people tight and stiff. All muscles shorten when they contract and lengthen when they relax. If muscle appears to lengthen due to training, this indicates a loss of skeletal muscle tissue. Obviously, this is not what trainees are looking for. If Pilates made muscles longer, this would mean that with prolonged Pilates training, your muscles would continue to get longer. Eventually, you wouldn't be able to move your joints due to increased slack.

Do Pilates exercises offer more exercises than weight training does?

ANSWER: There are many, many different exercises possible with free weights. If variety is so important to Pilates advocates, they should incorporate some other modes of weight training into their programs.

INVESTIGATION: Pilates boasts that it includes more than 2,000 exercises. According to Pilates proponents, Pilates features much more variety than is offered with weight training. Proponents who make these claims obviously haven't done much weight training. Weight training includes barbells, dumbbells, kettlebells, clubbells, nonconforming objects, medicine balls—and so on. The variety offered by Pilates pales in comparison with that offered by weight training.

How do Pilates exercises compare with weight training?

ANSWER: Heavy weight training, done in a proper manner, enhances back strength (in healthy trainees). Pilates exercises, performed in conjunction with other training modes, can offer benefits for some people. Although different from weight training, Pilates is still a form of resistance training.

INVESTIGATION: Some Pilates advocates claim that Pilates corrects muscle imbalances, heals bad backs, and realigns the body. Weight training, they say, causes muscle imbalances and is bad for back health. Actually, both properly designed Pilates programs (other than Pilates resistance training) and properly designed weight-training programs can be used to correct muscle imbalances, heal bad backs, and realign the body. Conversely, both programs can be detrimental if used incorrectly. It is hard to argue with the fact that power lifters, strongmen, and Olympic weightlifters possess enormous back strength, stability, and power—yet they all lift very heavy weights.

A study published in 2000 in the *International Journal of Sports Medicine* investigated the lumbar spine of a world record holder in the squat lift. The investigation revealed the highest bone mineral density reported to date (at that time). An MRI showed normal alignment and no evidence of disc hernia or compressive disc disease.

Do sports science journals provide objective, unbiased information?

ANSWER: Sports science journals are the best sources of information available. But they are not perfect and should be critically analyzed. Also, there are different types of scientific research, with different research methods. In order to analyze scientific research critically, it's important to understand the different methods.

INVESTIGATION: The most reliable information available is derived from sports science journals. But this information is not error free. Much of the scientific research conducted in sports science is sponsored by companies or groups with a vested interest in the outcome. This may lead to discarding unwanted results or interpreting results in a manner that supports an outcome that is favorable to a company or group.

The peer review process is used by sports science journals to ensure the publication of objective, unbiased information. The problem with this is that it's hard to find objective, unbiased reviewers. Reviewers carry with them their own education, experience, and preconceived notions; all of these affect their objectivity. Their knowledge may also be limited on a particular subject matter. Also, reviewers are often busy with work and other projects, which limits the time they spend reviewing the information.

Do I need to undergo prescreen exercise testing before beginning an exercise program?

ANSWER: Under most circumstances, formal prescreen exercise testing is not mandatory, although it is recommended that you complete an extensive questionnaire before starting an exercise regimen. If you have a pre-existing medical condition, you should have a full examination before beginning an exercise regimen. If a trainer insists on administering exercise tests, don't be afraid to ask questions about the test. The trainer should appreciate your curiosity and be happy to answer your questions.

INVESTIGATION: A study published in 1989 in the *Annals of Internal Medicine* investigated the role of exercise testing in screening for coronary artery disease. The researchers concluded that the effect of exercise testing is too small to justify doing this procedure routinely in healthy persons. Stress tests often give false positives and have a low success rate in discovering "silent" heart disease. "Studies reveal that as few as 20% of subjects whose stress tests indicate possible heat disease actually have coronary artery disease," says Mel Siff.

Dr. Henry Solomon, of Cornell University Medical School, is the author of *The Exercise Myth* and suggests that stress testing can expose individuals to higher stress levels than they are used to in everyday life, thus stressing them unnecessarily.

Fitness professionals often administer a variety of exercise tests, although many of these tests are of minimal value and are conducted to generate extra money, not test fitness parameters. The "sit-and-reach" test is an example of these popular tests. The test is performed by reaching forward while sitting on the floor with legs extended in front of the body, toes pointing up and feet slightly apart, and with the soles of the feet against the base of a flat surface (a step or a reach box is often used). At the point of the greatest reach, the individual holds for a couple of seconds. The reach is then measured. This test is used to measure overall flexibility. But there is a big problem: it doesn't actually measure overall flexibility. Flexibility is movement plane specific, speed specific, and joint specific. The sit-and-reach test is a single movement that measures static flexibility in a single plane. To measure overall flexibility, a variety of tests are needed.

Is aerobic activity better than anaerobic activity for cardiac health?

ANSWER: Aerobic and anaerobic exercise can both be beneficial to cardiac health. The claim that aerobic exercise is better than anaerobic exercise for cardiac health is not supported by science. When considering cardiac health, more than one factor must be taken into account. It is well documented that longevity and cardiac health are influenced by multiple factors.

INVESTIGATION: Low-intensity aerobics can be beneficial for cardiac health, but is it the most beneficial form of exercise? Some have implied that in addition to improving cardiac health, aerobics can enhance longevity. The same people have indicated that anaerobic exercises have no benefits related to heart health.

The Harvard Alumni Health Study, published in 2000, examined the association between the intensity of physical activity and coronary heart disease (CHD) risk and the impact of other coronary risk factors. They followed 12,516 middle-aged and older men (mean age 57.7 years, range 39–88 years) from 1977 through 1993. At the end of the study, researchers concluded that total physical activity and vigorous activities showed the strongest reductions in CHD risk. Moderate and light activities, which may be less precisely measured, showed insignificant inverse associations with CHD risk.

In another study, Dr. Paffenbarger looked at two populations—Harvard University graduates (1998) who exercised in their leisure time and San Francisco longshoremen (1979) who exercised vigorously as part of their work. The study was conducted over many decades. He found that the risk of heart attack was less in longshoremen. Work done by longshoremen is strenuous and sporadic resistance activity. This is not similar to low-intensity aerobic activity. The evidence from this study seems to indicate that anaerobic training can have positive impacts on cardiac health. Keep in mind that this was a correlation—not causation—study. Factors other than activity could have influenced the findings.

Does heavy weight training increase muscle tension?

ANSWER: When working to increase muscle tension, you don't have to rely solely on heavy weight training. Nonweighted movements, such as plyometrics (exercises to increase explosive strength by stimulating the muscles with of a sudden stretch preceding any voluntary effort), jumping, and sprinting, can produce more tension in the muscles than heavy weight training.

INVESTIGATION: Increasing muscle tension is associated with increasing load (weight on the bar). There are factors other than load that affect muscle tension, including acceleration in the direction of the muscle, leverage relative to the joint involving the relevant muscle group, the elasticity of the connective tissues associated with the muscle, stretch reflexes, pliability, the involvement of other muscle groups, and the distribution of types of muscle fiber. Plyometrics, as well as various types of jumping and sprinting activities, have been shown to produce significant amounts of tension in the muscle.

Do advanced athletes need to warm up before exercising?

ANSWER: A proper warm-up is beneficial to anyone who exercises, whether beginner or advanced level. On the other hand, cool muscles have been shown to display less strength. When warming up before the workout, don't exhaust yourself. If you feel yourself getting tired and out of breath, rest. Don't perform excessive static stretching (holding stretches in a steady position) before training. This type of stretching can be detrimental to dynamic activity (activity that involves movement) and can induce fatigue and weaken your stretch reflex. A small bit of static stretching may not be bad before a dynamic workout, but for the most part, stick to dynamic range-of-motion stretching preworkout and static stretching postworkout.

INVESTIGATION: The purpose of the warm-up is to increase the functional potential of the body. The warm-up is divided into general and specific phases. For example, a general warm-up for boxing includes dynamic range-of-motion stretching (stretching while moving) and jumping rope. A specific warm-up for boxing includes movements that are associated with specific movement patterns, such as shadow boxing.

Practical implications regarding warm-ups:

- A muscle contracts more rapidly and more intensely the higher its temperature is, within its safe physiological range.
- The electrical activity of a muscle increases with rising body temperature and after stimulation.
- Increasing temperature locally increases strength, as measured by a dynamometer and by the amount of time a muscle can maintain a specific tension or perform a measured volume of work.
- Hot showers have been shown to increase isometric endurance as well as the speed of muscular contraction and endurance in cyclic work.

Are sport-specific exercise programs beneficial?

ANSWER: The primary goal of a sport-specific exercise program is to enhance performance in a particular sport. Programs that fail to recognize performance as the most important goal are not real sport-specific programs. Designers of authentic sport-specific programs realize that their exercise programs should not replace skill training, but simply augment it.

INVESTIGATION: Almost every gym I know of offers sport-specific programs—or at least, what they call sport-specific programs. The typical sport-specific program includes some free weight movements, maybe some speed training, and some exercises that mimic the movement of a particular sport. Very few of these programs address quickness, agility, anaerobic endurance, power, and so on. A sport-specific program should enhance the specific fitness qualities required in a particular sport. Many commercial gyms, personal trainers, and sports conditioning coaches fail in this endeavor.

Following is a list of some key factors to consider when designing a sport-specific program:

- Identify the most important qualities required to play the sport successfully.
- Identify the most important qualities required to play a specific position.
- Identify an individual's strengths and weaknesses.
- Identify the most common injuries that occur in that sport, as well as injuries most common in different positions.
- Identify movement patterns often performed in the sport and movement patterns of different positions in the sport.
- Identify primary energy systems used in the sport and energy systems used by different positions and individuals.

When designing a sport-specific program, it is imperative to identify and address the qualities mentioned in the preceding list. Unfortunately, poorly designed programs seem to be the norm. For example, many high school football programs don't incorporate agility work into their training. Yet agility—the ability to accelerate, decelerate, and rapidly change direction while maintaining balance—is a key attribute needed to succeed in football. Many boxers run 3 to 4 miles a day and perform minimal or no weight training. Running 3 to 4 miles a day develops the aerobic energy system, which plays a minor role in boxing. These are just two examples among the many examples of poor program design.

Are slow training movements more effective than rapid movements?

ANSWER: Emphasizing slow training movements is detrimental to physical conditioning, although for unhealthy trainees slow movements may be warranted on occasion. The majority of slow training advocates are attracted to this method because they believe it decreases the chances of injury. They have been persuaded that rapid training is injurious, due to large momentums generated, while slow training is the safe alternative. In reality, if the avoidance of large momentums is the objective, slow training proponents should refrain from any participation in sports due to the very rapid movements and large momentums that often occur.

INVESTIGATION: Slow training advocates claim that slow exercise speed minimizes momentum and maximizes muscle tension. This statement is incorrect. Momentum is defined as mass times velocity. Moving light loads quickly may generate large momentums; similarly, moving heavy loads slowly can generate large momentums. Ergonomic studies have shown that more low back pain and disability is produced by some form of relaxed sitting than by Olympic weightlifting, especially if spinal flexion of prolonged duration occurs. At slow speed or at rest, the body is always affected by gravity. A slow speed or no speed at all can be just as stressful and dangerous as high speed.

Slow training advocates contend that maximal strengthening and hypertrophy (muscular growth) occur with their methods. Scientific research, thousands of trainees, and I disagree. If you try to lift a heavy weight slowly, you won't be able to lift the weight. When trying to lift a heavy weight, it is important to think, *Explosion*. In attempting to lift the weight fast, more force is applied to the bar. Slow training methods are also detrimental to power production. Power is work divided by time. Power is a combination of speed and strength.

Is the motto "No pain, no gain" valid when working out?

ANSWER: Designing an exercise program based on the "No pain, no gain" mantra can result in excessive tiredness and soreness. Exercise is supposed to make you feel better, not tired and beat down all of the time. When exercise begins to affect everyday activities negatively, it's time to reevaluate your exercise program. An occasional "torture session" may not necessarily be a bad thing; it may improve mental toughness. But relying on extreme workouts on a regular basis leads to excessive physiological and psychological stress.

INVESTIGATION: "No pain, no gain" is a chant often heard in gyms around the country. The phrase is often seen on bumper stickers and T-shirts. The idea that a painful workout is necessary to create gains has been taken to the extreme. Some trainers and coaches thrive on making athletes sore or making them vomit. How much knowledge is required to design a workout that creates fatigue and severe discomfort? If fatigue and severe discomfort were the only requirements for a successful training regimen, you wouldn't need anything more than intense calisthenics.

Soreness is generally caused by overstress or by performing novel movements. Beginners often experience delayed-onset muscle soreness, which has nothing to do with the value of the exercise. If soreness were an indicator of quality workouts, high-level athletes would be sore all the time, which would detract from their sport skill training. There is no evidence that muscle soreness is necessary to induce hypertrophy (muscular growth) or maximal strength.

Should so-called dangerous exercises be avoided?

ANSWER: The possibility for injury always exists, no matter what type of exercises you do. So-called dangerous exercises offer a wide array of benefits to trainees and should not be completely avoided. To prevent injury, some of these movements require that extra attention be given to technique and, in some cases, require the supervision of a coach. With prolonged training, you are bound to suffer at least minor injuries, but with proper program design, these can be minimized.

INVESTIGATION: So-called dangerous exercises include squats, overhead presses, and dead lifts, to name a few. Various training authorities have suggested that these movements should be avoided due to a great potential for injury. They fail to mention that there is always a chance of injury with any type of exercise, whether it's a so-called dangerous exercise or not.

Common causes of injury include the following:
- defective equipment
- excessive exertion while ill or injured
- inadequate recovery time
- excessive loads
- excessive acceleration or deceleration
- excessive range of motion for a particular joint
- unsafe use of momentum
- inefficient patterns of movement
- inappropriate warming up or stretching
- excessive warming up, which results in fatigue
- lack of concentration while training
- trying too hard to keep up with a partner (often to impress others)

Are strong abdominals the most important aspect of fitness?

ANSWER: Total body fitness is determined by a multitude of factors; abdominal strength is only one factor. To strengthen the midsection adequately, trunk flexion, rotation, lateral flexion, trunk extension, and core stabilizer movements are required.

INVESTIGATION: The abdominal muscles are the most overemphasized muscle group in physical training. Many people are obsessed with seeing a "six-pack," which, in fact, is determined by a low body fat percentage and has little correlation with strength. Training to enhance midsection strength is often misguided. Training the midsection using thousands of repetitions does little to enhance maximal strength. Too much focus on trunk flexion movements (sit-ups) at the expense of rotational movements (twisting crunches), lateral flexion movements (side bends), and stabilization movements (planks) results in midsection imbalances. Too much emphasis on midsection movements can also lead to an imbalance in overall fitness. The average trainee places too much emphasis on abdominal training and neglects back training.

Here are some basic rules about abdominal and trunk exercises:
- Straight leg crunches greatly inhibit hip flexor stimulation.
- High-repetition abdominal training does little to strengthen the abdominals (maximal strength), although high reps may increase endurance.
- Hanging leg raises or knee raises are a poor abdominal movement unless performed with a pike movement.
- Do not neglect training the lower back.
- Lower backs are generally weak because they are not exercised, not because of weak abdominals.
- Lumbar stress and hip flexor activity increase when the legs are held or anchored.
- Beyond 30 degrees above horizontal, the abdominals become less active because the hip flexors become the prime movers.
- Abdominal training does not reduce fat around the waistline.
- Maximal sit-up repetitions are primarily a test of hip flexor endurance.

- Leg throwdowns can produce a large torque of the hips and great stress on the lumbar region.
- Side bends activate the side flexors (*quadratus lumborum*).
- Sucking in the abdominals does not enhance the quality of abdominal training (in fact, this technique can decrease stabilizer strength and be dangerous with some movements, such as heavy squatting).
- To strengthen the abdominals adequately, add resistance.
- The abdominals are just one body part. Do not neglect the remainder of the body.
- It is low body fat and extracellular fluid levels that primarily determine the six-pack (clearly defined midsection) look.
- The overwhelming majority of infomercial ab devices are ineffective. Don't waste your money.

Are exercise machines safer than free weights?

ANSWER: Machines and free weights both have dangers associated with their use. It's important that exercisers be aware of the potential dangers associated with both. There is insufficient evidence to state that one is more dangerous than the other.

INVESTIGATION: Some modern gyms are equipped with machines only (no free weights) on the basis of the claim that free weights are "too dangerous." This is erroneous, as both can pose risks.

Following are some considerations for using machines safely:

- Seated vertical pressing machines often cause trainees to lean forward from the hip and hyperextend the lumbar spine.
- Hack squat machines can impose excessive shearing forces on the knee and eliminate natural movement patterns.
- Lying inclined or vertical leg press machines often result in forced lumbar flexion. (This is a weak mechanical position for the back under

99

these circumstances; be careful to not excessively round the back when performing this movement.)

- Foot rests on seated vertical pressing machines are often in a position that makes it hard for you to stabilize yourself. Keep your feet on the ground if you are having difficulty stabilizing your body when placing your feet on the footrest.

- Most bench press machines require you to begin the movement from a mechanically weak position (bar at chest, which inhibits prestretch). This can be good if you are training at starting strength, trying to eliminate the stretch-shortening cycle (when the stretch precedes muscle contraction) or both.

- Pec decks almost always have you begin from a mechanically weak position, where your shoulders are starting from a position of extreme external rotation. Be cautious when using this machine; excessive external rotation can be damaging, especially for individuals with shoulder range-of-motion issues.

- When using standing calf raise machines, pay close attention to your lower back position. It is not unusual for a trainee to flex the lumbar spine and induce injury.

- Standing hip adduction/abduction machines that require you to pull or push the straightened leg against a loaded lever arm often result in excessive simultaneous spinal rotation or flexion/extension. This type of spinal action has a high potential to injure the lumbar spine.

- Smith machines, which guide the bar to slide upward on a fixed path, usually impose larger loads on the shoulders and wrists than standing or seated presses with free weights.

- Machines that require you to sit prevent you from using your hip, knee, and ankle joints to absorb shock. Holding the natural pelvic tilt becomes much harder. Spinal flexion or hyperextension occurs more easily and spinal stress becomes more likely. Pay close attention to spinal posture when performing seated or standing exercises using this machine.

- If a machine isolates a joint, there is a more concentrated stress on that particular joint (which, in some cases, is not good). When performing a leg extension, the hip joint is taken out of the movement, and thus a greater stress is placed on the knee joint.

- Using seated spinal twist machines often results in flexion of the lumbar spine while rotating. It can also result in excessive torsional loading on spinal ligaments. Be very careful if you choose to use this contraption. Better yet, don't use "the crippler." (You might be surprised at how many rehabilitation facilities own this piece of equipment, even though injury risk is high.)

Are strength and power the same thing?

ANSWER: Strength and power are not exactly the same thing. It is possible to be strong but not powerful, while being powerful almost always indicates at least relatively good strength.

INVESTIGATION: The terms *strength* and *power* are used interchangeably, which is not accurate. This can create confusion when considering how to train for strength or power. Strength is the application of force (push or pull), and there are different types of strength. Power is strength with speed. Technically, power is work (force X distance) divided by time. In many sports, power is more important than strength alone. At the same time, the development of maximum strength often leads to increases in power (particularly in beginners). But being strong does not necessarily mean being powerful.

The confusion of these terms becomes evident when we consider the sport of power lifting. When compared with weightlifting, the power lifts (squat, bench press, and dead lift) take longer to elevate a heavier weight a shorter distance, resulting in a relatively low power measurement. Power lifting was referred to as the odd lifts when competitions first began in the United States. At the same time, the British referred to these lifts as strength lifting (which is scientifically correct). Eventually, the sport came to be called power lifting.

Should women's fitness regimens be drastically different from men's?

ANSWER: Women can use the same exercises as men and train hard like men. Basically, the same training principles apply to both men and women.

INVESTIGATION: When a woman begins a fitness regimen, a couple of key issues need to be considered: anterior cruciate ligament (ACL) injuries and the "appearing ladylike" training mentality. Women competing in sports that involve jumping and pivoting are four to six times more likely to sustain an ACL injury than their male counterparts. Research indicates that possible causes of this higher incidence of ACL injury could be due to a number of factors, including the overdevelopment of quadriceps strength in relation to hamstring strength, a tight posterior chain, weak joints during certain phases of the menstrual cycle, inadequate landing, and a lack of agility training. All of these factors should be considered before beginning an exercise regimen. Be sure to begin slowly and progress at a reasonable pace to more intense workouts. Also, women sometimes feel uncomfortable seeming "unladylike" while working out, particularly in public settings. But you should sweat and make noise when you're training. You're in the gym to get results, which means hard work that might not be pretty.

Are certified fitness trainers highly qualified trainers?

ANSWER: A certified fitness trainer is not necessarily a highly qualified trainer. Unfortunately, most fitness trainer certifications are nothing more than paid endorsements. Whether a trainer is certified or not should be the least of your concerns when considering the quality of a trainer. There are many high-quality certified trainers and there are many high-quality noncertified trainers.

INVESTIGATION: When trying to find a good fitness trainer, a potential client should ask himself or herself the following questions. *What type of information does the trainer give to clients? What type of results have clients seen? How well are clients able to use the information on their own (without the trainer monitoring them)? Can the trainer provide references? Can the trainer supply answers to basic exercise and nutrition questions? Can the trainer offer evidence for any claims?* Good trainers know their limits. If they can't answer a question, they are honest and admit that. Good trainers give advice only about things they know about. And they do not state their opinions as facts, but as opinions. Finally, good trainers are usually first-rate motivators.

Does practice really "make perfect"?

ANSWER: Performing frequent workouts using good technique under stable conditions optimizes skill mastery. If the technique is practiced incorrectly, this leads to the development of incorrect movement patterns, and unlearning these patterns can be very difficult. The primary goal of technique training is to attain proper form, which— with sufficient repetition—becomes second nature. Imperfect practice makes imperfect performance. And (to be realistic) *nearly* perfect practice makes *nearly* perfect performance.

INVESTIGATION: Everybody knows that practice makes perfect, right? But this statement is an oversimplification. Practicing with incorrect technique can lead to the development of stubborn bad habits. It is debatable whether beginners should practice sport-specific skills in the absence of a coach. Beginners, especially in high-skill sports (such as Olympic weightlifting or boxing), are unlikely to have very good technique in the early stages of learning. If a coach is present, he or she can correct these technique flaws. The more a movement pattern is performed incorrectly, the harder it is to correct.

Stages of mastering technique:

Stage 1: The first stage of learning involves a very high excitation of the central nervous system. Usually, muscles are overused because they are tenser than necessary, extra movements are performed, and unnecessary muscle groups are recruited in the performance of a movement.

Stage 2: In the second stage, precision and economy of movement are increased. The metabolic cost of activity is lowered. The sequence of the excitation and inhibition of the central nervous system is formed.

Stage 3: In this stage, movements are more automatic. The athlete does not have to be verbally cued regarding proper technique. The technique becomes increasingly efficient. Economy of movement is greater than in stage 2.

Stage 4: In the fourth stage, the technique is sound. Now the technique can be performed well even under varying conditions (fatigue, noise, unfamiliar surroundings, and so on).

Is it necessary to exercise to lose weight?

ANSWER: Some people lose weight while exercising, some while dieting, and some use a combination of the two. The primary ingredient of weight loss is consuming fewer calories than maintenance level on a regular basis. However, to increase fitness levels, exercise is necessary. The best method of weight loss for most people is a combination of moderate exercise and moderate dieting.

INVESTIGATION: The National Center for Health Statistics shows that 68.7 percent of Americans are overweight, with a little more than 34 percent being obese and slightly less than 6 percent being "extremely obese." With the amount of money being invested in gym memberships, exercise equipment, and personal trainers, you would think that more people would be losing weight. But many people who have invested money in exercise equipment and gym memberships don't exercise on a regular basis. Others, who work out regularly, are still not losing weight.

Some gain weight when they exercise, and others drop significant amounts of weight when exercising. In general, exercise contributes to weight loss. If you aim to lose weight, focus on expending more calories than you consume.

Are kettlebells more effective than barbells?

ANSWER: Kettlebells have proven beneficial. They present a different stimulus than that of a barbell. Kettlebells are a wonderful addition to a comprehensive program, but—for most people—are not a replacement for barbells.

INVESTIGATION: I have been exercising with kettlebells for more than a decade. (I was using them when most people thought that they were a passing fad.) Times have changed and almost every gym you visit now has kettlebells. I know a few individuals who use only kettlebells in their training regimens—no dumbbells or barbells. Various companies manufacture kettlebells and offer kettlebell trainer certifications. The kettlebell craze is in full swing.

The original kettlebell, or *girya*, is a cast iron weight that looks like a bowling ball with a handle attached. The kettlebell and kettlebell sport lifting were developed in Russia. The first official Russian kettlebell competition took place in 1948. In the following years, kettlebell competitions became increasingly popular. In 1974, many Soviet republics recognized *girevoy* sport as "an ethnic sport." In 1985, the first USSR National Girevoy Sport Championship took place. The competition consisted of two movements. The power clean and jerk and the power snatch were used in competition. The movements were performed while counting the maximum number of repetitions that could be performed with each movement. Russian strongmen and wrestlers of the past attributed a great deal of their success to kettlebell training. Kettlebells were so popular in Russia that strongmen and weightlifters were called kettlebell men. Turn-of-the-twentieth-century German strongman Arthur Saxon included kettlebell movements in his training regimen. With time, kettlebells fell out of favor in the West. Kettlebells made a comeback in the early twenty-first century, and today they are more popular than ever.

Which is better, a kettlebell snatch or a barbell snatch? How about a kettlebell press or a barbell press? The answer to these questions is, It depends. It depends on training goals, level of fitness, training phase, space availability, and so on. Those are just two among many movements that can be performed with a barbell or kettlebell. I generally use kettlebells to train strength endurance and barbells for maximum strength and power, although from time to time I reverse roles and use kettlebells for strength and power and barbells for endurance.

Does high-intensity exercise increase appetite?

ANSWER: Based on my research and observations, high-intensity exercise generally decreases appetite and low-intensity exercise increases appetite.

INVESTIGATION: Low-intensity exercise may lead to increased appetite due to its ability to increase ghrelin, a hormone of gastric origin that has been shown to stimulate appetite and food intake. A study published in 2007 in *Regulatory Peptides* investigated the effect of exercise intensity and duration on ghrelin release and food intake in normal-weight subjects. The researchers concluded that "low- rather than high-intensity exercise stimulates ghrelin levels independent of exercise duration."

A study published in 1988 in *Medicine and Science in Sports and Exercise* investigated the acute effects of two exercise intensities, low and high, on appetite. The researchers concluded, "Exercise, while not decreasing food intake, does not appear to increase it, and the benefits of exercise for body fat reduction are not immediately offset by compensatory caloric intake." In other words, high-intensity or low-intensity exercise increases caloric expenditure and is beneficial to weight loss.

CHAPTER 3

FINDING THE RIGHT DIET FOR WEIGHT LOSS

Starting a new weight-loss program can be intimidating. There are so many questions and so many different answers. With so much conflicting advice, it's no wonder that people can be worried and discouraged before they even begin. In general, most people have similar questions, whether they are beginners or advanced exercisers. In this chapter, I highlight some factors to consider in deciding on a diet program. I also answer some of the questions that I have been asked most often in my years as a personal trainer.

Looking Past the Hype When Considering Different Diets

To optimize the effectiveness of a diet, many factors should be considered, including your level of activity, genotype, primary goals, metabolic abnormalities, past experiences with dieting, responses to meal frequency, psychological issues, convenience issues, food availability, and support systems. Many weight management programs are too generic and do not take these factors into consideration.

Should I Eat the Yolk?

An ineffective program might, for example, assume that its specific recommendations would apply to everyone (even with strenuous activity, sickness, a low-carbohydrate diet, metabolic disorders, very-low-calorie consumption, or some other variable).

Investigate Whether Scientific Information Is Accurate

When considering the science behind weight-loss programs, there are several things to remember. Reliable scientific information is derived from primary scientific research (original measurements and recordings performed by those conducting research in the field or a lab). When analyzing primary scientific research data, it's important to consider research design, how the results were extrapolated, who conducted the research, and who—if anyone—has a vested interest in the design or outcome (that is, does someone have something to gain or lose). It is not necessary to acquire an advanced understanding of research methodology, as this could take years, but even a basic understanding would be beneficial. You can learn the basics with a moderate time investment. There are a variety of websites and books dedicated to reading scientific research. Secondary research examines and analyzes primary research. Depending on the skill and biases of the reporter, secondary research can be good or bad.

When considering the advice given by a nutritionist, it's important to know if the advice is derived from current primary scientific data or is based on other sources—secondary, tertiary, testimonials, case studies, and so on. In most cases, the advice given is not derived directly from primary research. Some people who promote themselves as scientists don't actually examine the primary research data. Of course, that doesn't mean that their advice is wrong—it just means that they really don't know if it's wrong or if it's right.

Weight Loss Is Not the Only Measurement of Success

Weight loss comes in various forms (including fat, body proteins, water, toxins, glycogen, and mineral storage). Body composition can be important for health, performance, and physique. In addition to weight loss, measurements are important when determining the successfulness of a program and overall health. Don't rely on the scale alone to give you an accurate reading of your fitness.

Be Wary of Weight Management Programs That Push or Even Insist on Their Own Food or Supplements

Supplements can play a positive role in weight management, but they're not magic and their nutrition is not superior to the nutrition found in food. The word *supplement* means "to complement" the program, not "to replace" exercise or the nutrients found in food.

I'm not antisupplement, but I am antinonsense. Sometimes supplements are beneficial because they are more convenient and cheaper than food. If you need supplements to get the job done, go for it. However, packaged foods and massive quantities of supplements are not necessities for weight loss. A company that requires you to buy their supplements or food is not necessarily interested in your losing weight or upgrading your nutritional status.

Requirements of a Quality Diet

Many different diets lead to weight loss, physique enhancement, and a healthier body. In other words, many roads lead to the same place. If you can't stick to the diet, it won't be successful. The psychological aspect of dieting is often overlooked, but is crucial in determining success. Pick a diet that you can stick with. If you hate all of the foods included in the diet and you're really dreading beginning the diet—choose a different one. A quality diet takes the following into account:

- Adequate calories. (This matters whether you're consciously counting calories or not.)
- Essential nutrients.
- Individual likes and dislikes.
- Metabolic abnormalities.
- Occasional breaks. (You don't have to stick to the program 100 percent of the time to see the benefits.)

Frequently Asked Questions

I just started a new workout program, and am wondering how many days per week I need to work out. I am mainly concerned with weight loss.

There is no specific requirement regarding your workout schedule. You need to design an exercise regimen that will fit into your schedule. Exercise doesn't have to be torture. Find some type of regimen that you will actually follow. Don't try to follow a routine just because a friend or someone in a magazine suggests it. The most important predictor of your success is your adherence to the program. In other words, if you train with modest intensity for a moderate volume (that is, a moderate number of sets and repetitions) on a regular basis, you will probably see results. If, on a consistent basis, you eat fewer calories than you burn, you will drop weight. Approach diet with the same attitude that you have toward exercise. Find an eating plan you can follow.

General suggestions for beginners:
- Exercise 3 or 4 days per week.
- Perform weight training 2 or 3 days per week.
- Perform dynamic range-of-motion exercises before weight training, and static stretching exercises after weight training.
- Perform light to moderate aerobic activity 3 days per week.
- Start slow and don't overdo it.

If you are consistently sore, decrease the intensity or number of workouts per week.

Is it possible to eat all the meat and cheese I want and lose weight?

It depends on how much meat and cheese you eat. Many people have done well following diets that limit carbohydrates and have a moderate to large amount of meat and cheese. However, some people do not lose a significant amount of weight following this program. Generally, eating nonstarchy vegetables with the meat and cheese diet increases satiety. People who lose weight when eating all the meat and cheese they want, do so by consistently eating less than their calorie maintenance level.

I am not concerned about getting stronger, just about becoming fit. Do I need to lift weights?

Fitness requires the development of various qualities, including strength. If you are interested in total body fitness, I recommend some type of weight training. In the early stages of training, some beginners rely solely on body weight strength exercises, such as body weight squats, push-ups, planks, and so on. And for many people, light dumbbells are the only weight training equipment they need.

I weigh 150 pounds, I have just started working out, and I am trying to lose weight. How many calories should I eat?

It is hard to give an accurate suggestion based on body weight alone. That said, I have found that the *EZ Method* works for most people. Using this method, to find your calorie level, multiply your current body weight by 8 to 12 calories. The number you get will be the number of calories you should eat per day while on a weight-loss diet. Those individuals who are more active will multiply by higher numbers. If you are not losing weight, multiply by a lower number. I haven't met anyone trying to lose weight who needed to go much lower than 8.

Are there special foods I can eat that will help me lose weight?

There are no magic foods, but there are foods that are filling and low in calories, including high-fiber foods (fruits, vegetables, legumes, and grains), lean protein foods (lean beef, skinless turkey, and chicken breast), and potatoes. Other tips that may help you eat less include drinking water before eating a meal and eating more slowly.

I have tried almost every workout on the market, but I haven't found one that's effective. I currently weigh what I did six months ago. Any suggestions?

Ask yourself how many calories you are eating. Calories are just as important to consider as exercise when trying to lose weight. I recommend keeping a food log. Buy a calorie book and use it. Write down everything you eat, so you can get an idea of your caloric intake. You have to create a calorie deficit to lose weight. Some people exercise really hard but short-circuit their results because they eat too many calories. It is possible to consume small amounts of food but still be consuming too many calories. Not eating too much means not eating too many calories.

I like to work out every day. Is this too often?

That depends on your fitness level and your training goals. If you are training for a high-skill sport, you may need to do some training daily. Many high-level athletes train almost daily; however, properly planned layoffs from training are also important to prevent overtraining and are often required for mental rejuvenation. Working out daily is unnecessary and counterproductive for most people. The body needs exercise, but it also needs sufficient rest and recovery to maximize benefits. If you do decide to work out every day, be sure to alter the intensity (speed of movement and amount of weight used) and volume (sets and repetitions). It is not practical for most people to train at a high intensity or high volume for prolonged periods.

Is aerobic exercise necessary for weight loss?

No. Some of my leanest clients do zero aerobics. That doesn't mean, however, that aerobics are not beneficial or that they are not good for weight loss. Many people have lost lots of weight while following routines that rely primarily on aerobics. Aerobics can be used to increase cardiovascular health and produce a lower resting pulse. To be clear, aerobics can help with weight loss, but they are not a requirement. I generally recommend that general fitness enthusiasts perform moderate aerobic activity 3 or 4 times per week.

Why should most people drink milk?

Some people shouldn't drink milk. These are people who can't properly digest milk, or are allergic to it. For most people, however, milk is a great source of nutrition. Milk consumption is beneficial for bones and for building muscle. Most well-designed, randomized, and controlled trials indicate that milk is beneficial to both bone and muscle mass. If you're following a low-calorie diet, you may want to drink skim milk.

Is the glycemic index useful for weight loss? How about health?

The glycemic index (GI) has limited applicability for nondiabetic, active people who don't eat large amounts of single types of food in isolation. If you are a diabetic, are insulin resistant, or have a similar disorder, the GI should be considered. With most trials that lasted six months or longer, GI had no significant effect on body weight or body composition. Fit, active individuals shouldn't be overly concerned with the GI.

REFERENCES

Do high insulin levels cause obesity?
Freedman, M. R. et al. 2001. Popular diets: A scientific review. *Obesity Research* 9, Suppl. no. 1. (March).

Is it all right to eat fruit when dieting?
Hale, J. 2007. *The carbohydrate files 2nd edition.* Winchester, KY: MaxCondition Publishing.
—. 2007. *Knowledge and nonsense: The science of nutrition and exercise.* Winchester, KY: MaxCondition Publishing, 2007.

Is bottled water safer to drink than tap water?
Lalumandier, J. A., and L. W. Ayers. 2000. Fluoride and bacterial content of bottled water vs. tap water. *Archives of Family Medicine* 9 (3): 246–250.
Shermer, M. Bottled twaddle: Is bottled water tapped out? http://mail .colonial.net/~rpavlik/pavlikweb/pdf/handouts/water/bottledwater.pdf (accessed September 7, 2009).

Does bottled water taste better than tap water?
Penn & Teller. The truth about bottled water. http://www.youtube.com/ watch?v=JdvJOF-2mm0 (accessed September 7, 2009).

Shermer, M. Bottled twaddle: Is bottled water tapped out? http://mail
    .colonial.net/~rpavlik/pavlikweb/pdf/handouts/water/bottledwater.pdf
    (accessed September 7, 2009).

*Does it matter where calories come from? Or is a calorie a calorie, regardless
of its source?*
Hale, J. 2007. *Knowledge and nonsense: The science of nutrition and
    exercise.* Winchester, KY: MaxCondition Publishing.
McDonald, L. Is a calorie just a calorie? MaxCondition, http://www
    .maxcondition.com/page.php?11 (accessed December 7, 2009).

Are carbohydrates essential nutrients?
Hale, J. 2007. *The carbohydrate files 2nd edition.* Winchester, KY:
    MaxCondition Publishing.
——. 2007. *Knowledge and nonsense: The science of nutrition and exercise.*
    Winchester, KY: MaxCondition Publishing.

Can some people with lactose intolerance consume some dairy?
Hale, J. 2007. *The carbohydrate files 2nd edition.* Winchester, KY:
    MaxCondition Publishing.
——. 2007. *Knowledge and nonsense: The science of nutrition and exercise.*
    Winchester, KY: MaxCondition Publishing.

Given that coffee raises insulin levels acutely, should it be avoided?
Battram, D. S. et al. 2006. The glucose intolerance induced by caffeinated
    coffee ingestion is less pronounced than that due to alkaloid caffeine
    in men. *Journal of Nutrition* 136, no. 5 (May): 1276–80.
Beaty, J. Bodybuilding nutrition roundtable. Alan Argon.com. http://
    alanaragon.com/bodybuilding-nutrition-roundtable-alan-aragon-will-
    brink-jamie-hale-layne-norton.html (accessed September 10, 2009).
McGraw, J. 2004. *Brain and belief: An exploration of the human soul.* Del
    Mar, CA: Aegis Press.
Silvio, G., ed. 1993. *Caffeine, coffee and health.* New York: Raven Press.

Should I Eat the Yolk?

Does dietary fat have beneficial effects on testosterone levels?

Hamalainen, E. et al. 1984. Diet and serum sex hormones in healthy men. *Journal of Steroid Biochemistry* 20:459–64.

Raben, A. et al. 1992. Serum sex hormones and endurance performance after a lacto-ovo vegetarian and mixed diet. *Medicine and Science in Sports and Exercise* 24:1290–97.

Can people with hypothyroidism lose weight?

Hale, J. 2007. *Knowledge and nonsense: The science of nutrition and exercise.* Winchester, KY: MaxCondition Publishing.

Does eating specific types of foods together cause weight gain?

Beaty, J. Bodybuilding nutrition roundtable. Alan Aragon.com. http://alanaragon.com/bodybuilding-nutrition-roundtable-alan-aragon-will-brink-jamie-hale-layne-norton.html (accessed September 10, 2009).

Golay, A. et al. 2000. Similar weight loss with low-energy food combining or balanced diets. *International Journal of Obesity* 24 (4): 492–96.

Does eating grapefruit speed up fat loss?

Ballard, T. et al. 2006. Naringin does not alter caffeine pharmacokinetics, energy expenditure, or cardiovascular haemodynamics in humans following caffeine consumption. *Clinical and Experimental Pharmacology & Physiology* 33, no. 4 (April): 310–14.

Beaty, J. Bodybuilder nutrition roundtable. Alan Aragon.com. http://alanaragon.com/bodybuilding-nutrition-roundtable-alan-aragon-will-brink-jamie-hale-layne-norton.html (accessed September 10, 2009).

Do cortisol blockers, such as Relacore, cause weight loss?

Fichter, M. M. et al. 1986. *Psychiatry Research* 17, no. 1 (January): 61–72.

Are high-protein diets bad for bone health?

Heaney, R. P. et al. 1982. Effects of nitrogen, phosphorus, and caffeine on calcium balance in women. *Journal of Laboratory and Clinical Medicine* 99:46–55.

Heaney, R. 1999. Protein intake and bone health: The influence of belief systems and the conduct of nutritional science. *American Journal of Clinical Nutrition* 73, no. 1 (January): 5–6.

Katz, T. B. How to prevent osteoporosis. TBK Fitness. http://www.tbkfitness .org/osteoporosis.html (accessed September 11, 2009).

Do high-protein diets increase the risk of coronary heart disease (CHD)?
Hale, J. 2006. *Protein essentials.* Winchester, KY: MaxCondition Publishing.

Li, D. et al. 2005. Lean meat and heart health. *Asia Pacific Journal of Clinical Nutrition* 14 (2): 113–9.

Are high-protein diets are bad for the kidneys?
Hale, J. 2006. *Protein essentials.* Winchester, KY: MaxCondition Publishing.

Martin, W. F. et al. 2005. Dietary protein intake and renal function. *Nutrition and Metabolism* 2:25.

Should I eat only low glycemic index carbohydrates when trying to lose weight?
Hale, J. 2007. *The carbohydrate files 2nd edition.* Winchester, KY: MaxCondition Publishing.

——. Sport nutrition's best. MaxCondition. http://maxcondition.com/page .php?143 (accessed September 11, 2009).

Raatz, S. K. et al. 2005. Reduced glycemic index and glycemic load diets do not increase the effects of energy restriction on weight loss and insulin sensitivity in obese men and women. *Journal of Nutrition* 135 (10): 2387–91.

Raben, A. et al. 2002. Should obese patients be counseled to follow a low–glycemic index diet? *Obesity Reviews* 3 (4): 245–56.

To maximize weight loss, should I eat small amounts every two to three hours?
Bellisle, F. et al. 1997. Meal frequency and energy balance. *British Journal of Nutrition* 77 (1): S57–70.

Wolfram, G. et al. 1987. Thermogenesis in humans after varying meal time frequency. *Annals of Nutrition and Metabolism* 31 (2): 88–97.

Are dietary supplements necessary?
Lesser, L. et al. 2007. Relationship between funding source and conclusion among nutrition-related scientific articles. *PLoS Medicine* 4, no. 1 (January): e5.
Tipton, K. D. and O. C. Witard. 2007. Protein requirements and recommendations for athletes: Relevance of ivory tower arguments for practical recommendations. *Clinics in Sports Medicine*, 2007.

Is it okay to eat dairy when trying to lose weight?
Beaty, J. Bodybuilding nutrition roundtable. Alan Aragon.com. http://alanaragon.com/bodybuilding-nutrition-roundtable-alan-aragon-will-brink-jamie-hale-layne-norton.html (accessed September 10, 2009).
Hale, J. 2007. *Knowledge and nonsense: The science of nutrition and exercise.* Winchester, KY: MaxCondition Publishing.
——. Sport nutrition's best. MaxCondition. http://maxcondition.com/page.php?143 (accessed September 11, 2009).

Are low-carbohydrate diets bad for the brain?
Klepper, J. et al. 2003. The ketogenic diet in German-speaking countries: Update. Essen, Germany: *Universitats-Kinderklinik Essen.*
Reger, M. A. et al. 2004. Effects of betahydroxybutyrate on cognition in memory-impaired adults. *Neurobiology of Aging* 25 (3): 311–14.
Veech, R. L. 2004. The therapeutic implications of ketone bodies: The effects of ketone bodies in pathological conditions: Ketosis, ketogenic diet, redox states, insulin resistance, and mitochondrial metabolism. *Prostaglandins, Leukotrienes and Essential Fatty Acids* 70 (3): 309–19. Review.

Do low-carbohydrate diets lead to weight loss?

Alford, B. B. et al. 1990. The effects of variations in carbohydrate, protein, and fat content of the diet upon weight loss, blood values, and nutrient intake of adult obese women. *Journal of the American Dietetic Association* 90:534–40.

Freedman, M. R. et al. 2001. Popular diets: A scientific review. *Obesity Research* 9, Suppl. no. 1 (March).

Are the Recommended Dietary Allowances (RDA) protein guidelines sufficient for athletes?

Champe, P. C. et al. 2005. *Lippincott's Illustrated Reviews: Biochemistry.* 3rd ed. Philadelphia: Lippincott Williams and Wilkins.

Layman, D. K. 2009. Dietary guidelines should reflect new understandings about adult protein needs. *Nutrition and Metabolism* 6 (12).

Lemon, P. et al. 1998. Effects of exercise on dietary protein requirements. *International Journal of Sports Nutrition* 8 (4): 426–47.

Lucas, M. and C. J. Heiss. 2005. Protein needs of older adults engaged in resistance training: A review. *Journal of Aging and Physical Activity* 13 (2): 223–36.

Does eating sugar cause obesity?

Hale, J. 2007. *Knowledge and nonsense: The science of nutrition and exercise.* Winchester, KY: MaxCondition Publishing.

Are sweet potatoes more nutritious than white potatoes?

Aragon, A. 2007. *Girth control: The science of fat loss and weight gain.* Los Angeles, CA: Alan Aragon.

Mendosa, D. The satiety index rankings. Mendosa.com. http://www.mendosa.com/satrank.htm (accessed September 14, 2009).

Should I Eat the Yolk?

Should I eat the egg yolk?

Fernandez, M. L. 2006. Dietary cholesterol provided by eggs and plasma lipoproteins in healthy populations. *Current Opinion in Clinical Nutrition and Metabolic Care* 9, no. 1 (January): 8–12.

Greene, C. M. et al. 2005. Maintenance of LDL cholesterol: HDL cholesterol ratio in elderly population given a dietary cholesterol challenge. *Journal of Nutrition* 135, no. 12 (December): 2793–98.

Kritchevsky, S. B. 2004. A review of scientific research and recommendations regarding eggs. *Journal of the American College of Nutrition* 6, Suppl. (December 23): S596–S600.

Is the artificial sweetener sucralose unhealthy?

Baird, I. M. et al. 2000. Repeated dose study of sucralose in human subjects. *Food Chemical Toxicology* 38, Suppl. no. 2:S123–29.

Bigal, M. E. and A. V. Krymchantowski. 2006. Migraine triggered by sucralose, a case report. *Headache* 46 (3): 515–57.

Hale, J. 2007. *Knowledge and nonsense: The science of nutrition and exercise.* Winchester, KY: MaxCondition Publishing.

Grotz, V. L. et al. 2003. Lack of effect of sucralose on glucose homeostasis in subjects with type 2 diabetes. *Journal of the American Dietetic Association* 103 (12): 1607–12.

Do I have to avoid junk food completely to be lean?

Weaver, C. Down size me. http://chazzweaver.com/site/projects/down-size-me (accessed September 14, 2009).

Is organic food better for your health than conventional food?

Sil Dangour, A. D. et al. 2009. Nutritional quality of organic foods: A systematic review. *American Journal of Clinical Nutrition* 90:680–85.

Silver, L. M. 2006. *Challenging Nature.* New York: HarperCollins.

Whole Foods Market. 2005. *Whole Foods Market organic trend tracker.* Austin, TX: Whole Foods Market.

Winter, C. K. and S. F. Davis. 2006. Organic foods. *Journal of Food Science* 71 (9).

Does drinking oxygenated water enhance exercise performance?
Leibetseder, V. et al. 2006. Does oxygenated water support aerobic performance and lactate kinetics? *International Journal of Sports Medicine* 27:232–35.

Is a high-fiber diet recommended for everyone?
Hale, J. 2007. *The carbohydrate files 2nd edition.* Winchester, KY: MaxCondition Publishing.
——. 2007. *Knowledge and nonsense: The science of nutrition and exercise.* Winchester, KY: MaxCondition Publishing.

Is consuming soy good for your health?
Sacks, F. M. et al. 2006. Soy protein, isoflavones, and cardiovascular health: An American Heart Association science advisory for professionals from the Nutrition Committee. *Circulation* 113, no. 7 (February 21): 1034–44.
Taku, K. et al. 2007. Soy isoflavones lower serum total and LDL cholesterol in humans: A meta-analysis of 11 randomized controlled trials. *American Journal of Clinical Nutrition* 85 (4): 1148–56.
Zhan, S. and S. C. Ho. 2005. Meta-analysis of the effects of soy protein containing isoflavones on the lipid profile. *American Journal of Clinical Nutrition* 81 (2): 397–408.

Are dietary carbohydrates more beneficial than protein for endurance athletes?
Lemon, P. et al. 1998. Effects of exercise on dietary protein requirements. *International Journal of Sports Nutrition* 8 (4): 426–47.
Tarnopolsky, M. A. et al. 1988. Influence of protein intake and training status on nitrogen balance and lean body mass. *Journal of Applied Physiology* 64:187–93.

Should I Eat the Yolk?

Do sugar alcohols have an effect on blood sugar?

Bernstein, R. K. 2003. *Dr. Bernstein's Diabetes Solution: The Complete Guide to Achieving Normal Blood Sugars.* Revised ed. Boston, MA: Little, Brown and Company.

Livesey, G. 2003. Health potential of polyols as sugar replacers, with emphasis of low glycemic properties. *Nutrition Research Reviews* 16:163–91.

Mendosa, D. Net carbs: Can you really exclude sugar alcohols, glycerin, polydextrose, and fiber? Mendosa.com. http://mendosa.com/netcarbs.htm (accessed September 15, 2009).

Does carbohydrate loading enhance athletic performance?

Andrews, J. L. et al. 2003. Carbohydrate loading & supplementation in endurance-trained women runners. *Journal of Applied Physiology* 95:584–90.

Bassau, V. A. et al. 2002. Carbohydrate loading in human muscle: An improved 1-day protocol. *European Journal of Applied Physiology* 87, no. 3 (July): 290–95.

Burke et al. 2000. Carbohydrate loading failed to improve 100-km cycling performance in a placebo-controlled trial. *Journal of Applied Physiology* 88:1284–90.

Fairchild, T. J. et al. 2002. Rapid carbohydrate loading after a short bout of near maximal-intensity exercise. *Medicine and Science in Sports and Exercise* 34 (6): 980–86.

McDonald, L. 1998. *The Ketogenic Diet: A Complete Guide for the Dieter and Practitioner.* Austin, TX: Lyle McDonald.

Wilmore, J. H. et al. 1994. *Physiology of Sport and Exercise.* Champaign, IL: Human Kinetics.

Do excess carbohydrates in the diet turn into excess body fat?

Hellerstein, M. K. 1999. De novo lipogenesis in humans: metabolic and regulatory aspects. *European Journal of Clinical Nutrition* 53, Suppl. no. 1:S53–55.

McDevitt, R. M. et al. 2001. De novo lipogenesis during controlled overfeeding with sucrose or glucose in lean and obese women. *American Journal of Clinical Nutrition* 74(6): 737–46.

Does calcium intake enhance weight loss?

Gunther, C. W. et al. 2005. Dairy products do not lead to alterations in body weight or fat mass in young women in a 1-y intervention. *American Journal of Clinical Nutrition* 81 (4): 751–56.

Lorenzen, J. K. et al. 2006. Calcium supplementation for 1-y does not reduce body weight or fat mass in young girls. *American Journal of Clinical Nutrition* 83 (1): 18–23.

Shapses, S. A. et al. 2004. Effect of calcium supplementation on weight and fat loss in women. *Journal of Clinical Endocrinology and Metabolism* 89 (2): 632–7.

Do I really need to drink at least 8 glasses of water a day?

Grandjean, A. C. et al. 2000. The effect of caffeinated, non-caffeinated, caloric and non-caloric beverages on hydration. *Journal of the American College of Nutrition* 19 (5): 591–600.

Hale, J. 2007. *Knowledge and nonsense: The science of nutrition and exercise.* Winchester, KY: MaxCondition Publishing.

Valtin, H. 2002. "Drink at least eight glasses of water a day." Really? Is there scientific evidence for "8 x 8"? *American Journal of Physiology* 283, no. 5 (August): 993–1004.

Should athletes drink as much water as they can tolerate?

Burke, L. M. 2006. Fluid guidelines for sport: Interview with Professor Tim Noakes. *International Journal of Sport Nutrition and Exercise Metabolism* 16:644–52.

Noakes, T. 2007. Drinking guidelines for exercise: What evidence is there that athletes should drink "as much as tolerable," to replace the weigh lost during exercise or "ad libitum"? *Journal of Sports Sciences* 25:781–96.

Should I Eat the Yolk?

Can I eat late in the evening if I am trying to lose weight?
Hale, J. 2007. *Knowledge and nonsense: The science of nutrition and exercise.* Winchester, KY: MaxCondition Publishing.

Is weight loss slowed by not eating enough?
Owen, O. E. et al. 1998. Protein, fat, and carbohydrate requirements during starvation: anaplerosis and cataplerosis. *American Journal of Clinical Nutrition* 68:12–34.

Does alcohol consumption cause fat gain?
Sonko, B. J. et al. 1994. Effect of alcohol on postmeal fat storage. *American Journal of Clinical Nutrition* 59:619–25.

Are antioxidants good for my health?
Endemann, G. 2002. *Fat is not the enemy.* Tarentum, PA: Word Association Publishers.
Grodstein, F. et al. 2003. High-dose antioxidant supplements and cognitive function in community-dwelling elderly women. *American Journal of Clinical Nutrition* 77 (4): 762–63.
Kang, J. H. et al. 2006. A randomized trial of vitamin E supplementation and cognitive function in women. *Archives of Internal Medicine* 166 (22): 2433–34.
Omenn G. et al. 1996. Effects of a combination of beta-carotene and vitamin A on lung cancer and cardiovascular disease. *New England Journal of Medicine* 334 (18): 1150–55.

Is homeopathy an effective treatment for health problems?
Hill, C. and F. Doyon. 1990. Review of randomized trials of homeopathy. *Revue d'Epidemiologie et de Sante Publique* 38 (2): 139–47.
Kleijnen, J. et al. 1991. Clinical trials of homeopathy. *British Medical Journal* 302 (6772): 316–23.

National Council Against Health Fraud, Inc. NCAHF position paper on homeopathy. http://www.ncahf.org/pp/homeop.html (accessed September 18, 2009).

Shang, A. et al. 2005. Are the clinical effects of homeopathy placebo effects? Comparative study of placebo-controlled trials of homeopathy and allopathy. *Lancet* 366 (9487): 726–32.

Wagner, M. W. 2002. Is homeopathy "new science" or "new age"? Homeowatch. http://www.homeowatch.org/articles/wagner.html (accessed September 18, 2009).

Is sodium bad for my health?

Franco, V. and S. Oparil. 2006. Salt sensitivity, a determinant of blood pressure, cardiovascular disease and survival. *Journal of the American College of Nutrition* 25 (3): 247S–255S.

Gonzalez, A. O. et al. 1998. Salt sensitivity: concept and pathogenesis. *Diabetes Research and Clinical Practice* 39 (April): S15–S26,

Is aspartame bad for my health?

Hale, J. *Nutrition: fact or fiction.* PowerPoint Presentation.

Henkel, J. 2004. Sugar substitutes: Americans opt for sweeteners and lite. U.S. Food and Drug Administration. http://web.archive.org/web/20071214170430/www.fda.gov/fdac/features/1999/699_sugar.html (accessed September 19, 2009).

Is high-fructose corn syrup bad for my health?

Drewnowski, A. and F. Bellisle. 2007. Liquid calories, sugar, and body weight. *American Journal of Clinical Nutrition* 85 (3): 651–61.

Science Blog. Scientists say consumers confused about sugars. http://www.scienceblog.com/cms/scientists-say-consumers-confused-about-sugars-21934.html (accessed September 19, 2009).

White, J. S. 2008. Weak association between sweeteners or sweetened beverages and diabetes. *Journal of Nutrition* 138 (January):138.

Should I Eat the Yolk?

Is it possible to lose stubborn body fat?
Hale, J. 2007. *Knowledge and nonsense: The science of nutrition and exercise.* Winchester, KY: MaxCondition Publishing.
McDonald, L. 2003. *The Ultimate Diet 2.0.* Austin, TX: Lyle McDonald.

Will gaining muscle speed up my metabolism?
Hale, J. 2007. *Knowledge and nonsense: The science of nutrition and exercise.* Winchester, KY: MaxCondition Publishing.
McClave, S. A. and H. L. Snider. 2001. Dissecting the energy needs of the body. *Current Opinion in Clinical Nutrition and Metabolic Care* 4:143–47.

Will performing sit-ups shrink my waistline?
Aragon, A. 2007. *Girth control: The science of fat loss and weight gain.* Los Angeles, CA: Alan Aragon.

Will exercise get rid of cellulite?
Hale, J. 2007. *Knowledge and nonsense: The science of nutrition and exercise.* Winchester, KY: MaxCondition Publishing.
Rock, G. Myths exposed. Next Fitness Evolution. http://www.nextfitnessevolution.com (accessed November 1, 2007).

Will my muscle turn to fat if I stop weight training?
Siff, M. 2000. *Facts and fallacies of fitness.* Denver, Co: Mel Siff.
——. 2000. *Supertraining.* Denver, CO: Mel Siff.

If I train hard enough will I look like a pro bodybuilder?
Hale, J. 2007. *Knowledge and nonsense: The science of nutrition and exercise.* Winchester, KY: MaxCondition Publishing.
Siff, M. 2000. *Facts and fallacies of fitness.* Denver, Co: Mel Siff.

Are hanging leg raises a good exercise for the abdominals?
Hale, J. Ab training season. MaxCondition. http://www.maxcondition.com/page.php?59 (accessed December 10, 2009).

——. 2003. Examining the rules of fitness. http://dolfzine.com/page596.htm (site now discontinued).

——. 2000. *Optimum physique*. Winchester, KY: Jamie Hale.

Siff, M. 2000. *Facts and fallacies of fitness*. Denver, CO: Mel Siff.

Is weight training safe for children?

Drechsler, A. 1998. *The weightlifting encyclopedia: A guide to world class performance*. Whitestone, NY: A Is A Communications.

Hale, J. 2000. *Optimum physique*. Winchester, KY: Jamie Hale.

——. Young athletes and weight training. MaxCondition. http://www .maxcondition.com/page.php?51 (accessed December 10, 2009).

Siff, M. 2000. *Facts and fallacies of fitness*. Denver, CO: Mel Siff.

Are seated exercises safer than standing ones?

Hale, J. 2003. Examining the rules of fitness. http://dolfzine.com/page596 .htm (site now discontinued).

Siff, M. 2000. *Facts and fallacies of fitness*. Denver, CO: Mel Siff.

Will wearing a lifting belt weaken my midsection?

Siff, M. 2000. *Facts and fallacies of fitness*. Denver, CO: Mel Siff.

Are knee extensions more effective than squats for knee rehabilitation?

Hale, J. 2003. Examining the rules of fitness. http://dolfzine.com/page596 .htm (site now discontinued).

Siff, M. 2000. *Facts and fallacies of fitness*. Denver, CO: Mel Siff.

Is low-intensity, long-duration aerobics the best exercise for fat loss?

Aragon, A. 2006. Myths under the microscope part 1: The low intensity fat burning zone. Alan Aragon.com. http://alanaragon.com/myths-under-the-microscope-the-fat-burning-zone-fasted-cardio.html (accessed December 10, 2009).

Melanson, E. L. et al. 2002. Effect of exercise intensity on 24-h energy expenditure and nutrient oxidation. *Journal of Applied Physiology* 92, no. 3 (March): 1045–52.

Should I Eat the Yolk?

Saris, W. H. and P. Schrauwen. 2004. Substrate oxidation differences between high and low-intensity exercise are compensated over 24 hours in obese men. *International Journal of Obesity Related Metabolic Disorders* 28 (6): 759–65.

Does wearing strength shoes increase strength?
Cook, S. D. et al. 1993. Development of lower leg strength and flexibility with the strength shoe. *American Journal of Sports Medicine* 21 (3): 445–48.

Does wearing strength shoes increase flexibility?
Cook, S. D. et al. 1993. Development of lower leg strength and flexibility with the strength shoe. *American Journal of Sports Medicine* 21 (3): 445–48.

To gain muscle, must I do 3 sets of 10 repetitions of each exercise?
Moore, D. Work. http://hypertrophy-research.com/phpBB/viewtopic .php?t=8 (accessed November 1, 2007; site now discontinued).
Siff, M. 2000. *Facts and fallacies of fitness.* Denver, CO: Mel Siff.

Will high repetition weight training make me lean?
Zelasko, C. J. 1995. Exercise for weight loss: What are the effects? *Journal of the American Dietetic Association* 95, no. 12 (December): 1414–47.

Is it dangerous to lock the knees while exercising?
Hale, J. 2007. *Knowledge and nonsense: The science of nutrition and exercise.* Winchester, KY: MaxCondition Publishing.
Siff, M. 2000. *Facts and fallacies of fitness.* Denver, CO: Mel Siff.

Should I avoid back exercises if I have back problems?
Hale, J. 2007. *Knowledge and nonsense: The science of nutrition and exercise.* Winchester, KY: MaxCondition Publishing.
Siff, M. 2000. *Facts and fallacies of fitness.* Denver, CO: Mel Siff.

Is aerobic exercise recommended for all athletes?

Barros, R. Re: VO2 max of sprinters? E-mail to Yahoo.com mailing list.
supertraining@yahoogroups.com (accessed November 19, 2001).

Hatfield, F. C. 1993. *Fitness: The complete guide*. 2nd ed. Santa Barbara, CA:
The International Sports Sciences Association.

Siff, M. 2000. *Facts and fallacies of fitness*. Denver, CO: Mel Siff.

Is circuit training the best way to maximize fitness levels?

Gym Jones. Schedule—April 18, 2007. http://www.gymjones.com/schedule
.php?date=20070418 (accessed September 24, 2009).

Siff, M. 2000. *Supertraining*. Denver, CO: Mel Siff.

Will heavy weight training make me bulky?

Siff, M. 2000. *Facts and fallacies of fitness*. Denver, CO: Mel Siff.

——. 2000. *Supertraining*. Denver, CO: Mel Siff.

Will heavy weight training make me slow?

Drechsler, A. 1998. *The weightlifting encyclopedia: A guide to world class
performance*. Whitestone, NY: A Is A Communications.

Hale, J. 2003. Examining the rules of fitness. http://dolfzine.com/page596
.htm (site now discontinued).

Siff, M. 2000. *Supertraining*. Denver, CO: Mel Siff.

Does heavy weight training decrease flexibility?

Drechsler, A. 1998. *The weightlifting encyclopedia: A guide to world class
performance*. Whitestone, NY: A Is A Communications.

Newton, H. 2002. *Explosive lifting for sports*. Champaign, IL: Human
Kinetics.

USA Weightlifting. 1991. *USA club coach manual*. Colorado Springs, CO:
USA Weightlifting.

Do big muscles equal big strength?

Siff, M. 2000. *Supertraining*. Denver, CO: Mel Siff.

Should I Eat the Yolk?

Is light weight training safer than heavy weight training?
Hale, J. Machine hoopla. MaxCondition. http://www.maxcondition.com/
  page.php?50 (accessed December 10, 2009).
Siff, M. 2000. *Facts and fallacies of fitness.* Denver, CO: Mel Siff.

Is projecting the knees over the toes while exercising dangerous to the knees?
Siff, M. 2000. *Facts and fallacies of fitness.* Denver, CO: Mel Siff.

Should I pull in my stomach during exercise?
Siff, M. 2000. *Facts and fallacies of fitness.* Denver, CO: Mel Siff.
Zatsiorsky, V. 1995. *Science and practice of strength training.* Champaigne,
  IL: Human Kinetics.

Are standing dumbbell flies a good exercise for the chest?
Hale, J. 2007. *Knowledge and nonsense: The science of nutrition and
  exercise.* Winchester, KY: MaxCondition Publishing.
Siff, M. 2000. *Facts and fallacies of fitness.* Denver, CO: Mel Siff.

Are "good mornings," a lower back exercise, dangerous?
Zatsiorsky, V. 1995. *Science and practice of strength training.* Champaigne,
  IL: Human Kinetics.

Are squats better for the glutes than lunges are?
Hale, J. 2007. *Knowledge and nonsense: The science of nutrition and
  exercise.* Winchester, KY: MaxCondition Publishing.
Siff, M. 2000. *Facts and fallacies of fitness.* Denver, CO: Mel Siff.

Is it safer to use a suspended walking machine than to walk or run?
Hale, J. 2000. Machine hoopla. MaxCondition. http://www.maxcondition
  .com/page.php?50 (accessed December 10, 2009).
Siff, M. 2000. *Facts and fallacies of fitness.* Denver, CO: Mel Siff.

Do lying leg-press machines, or leg sleds, train the legs without stressing the back?

Hale, J. 2000. Machine hoopla. MaxCondition. http://www.maxcondition
.com/page.php?50 (accessed December 10, 2009).

Siff, M. 2000. *Facts and fallacies of fitness.* Denver, CO: Mel Siff.

Do machine exercises provide stress the same way as their free weight equivalents?

Hale, J. 2003. Examining the rules of fitness. http://dolfzine.com/page596
.htm (site now discontinued).

——. 2000. Machine hoopla. MaxCondition. http://www.maxcondition.com/
page.php?50 (accessed December 10, 2009).

Siff, M. 2000. *Facts and fallacies of fitness.* Denver, CO: Mel Siff.

Does being lean mean I am fit?

Hale, J. 2007. *Knowledge and nonsense: The science of nutrition and
exercise.* Winchester, KY: MaxCondition Publishing.

Can Pilates exercises lengthen my muscles?

Hale, J. Pilates magic. http://www.elitefts.com/documents/pilates_magic
.htm (accessed December 10, 2009).

Siff, M. 2000. *Facts and fallacies of fitness.* Denver, CO: Mel Siff.

Do Pilates exercises offer more exercise than weight training does?

Hale, J. Pilates magic. http://www.elitefts.com/documents/pilates_magic
.htm (accessed December 10, 2009).

Siff, M. 2000. *Facts and fallacies of fitness.* Denver, CO: Mel Siff.

How do Pilates exercises compare to weight training?

Dickerman, R. D. et al. 2000. The upper range of lumbar spine bone mineral
density. *International Journal of Sports Medicine* 21:469–70.

Hale, J. Pilates magic. http://www.elitefts.com/documents/pilates_magic
.htm (accessed December 10, 2009).

Siff, M. 2000. *Facts and fallacies of fitness.* Denver, CO: Mel Siff.

Should I Eat the Yolk?

Do sports science journals provide objective, unbiased information?
Aragon, A. 2007. *Girth control: The science of fat loss and weight gain.*
    Winchester, KY: Alan Aragon.
Siff, M. 2000. *Facts and fallacies of fitness.* Denver, CO: Mel Siff.

Do I need to undergo prescreen exercise testing before beginning an exercise program?
Siff, M. 2000. *Facts and fallacies of fitness.* Denver, CO: Mel Siff.
Sox, H. C., Jr. et al. 1989. The role of exercise testing in screening for
    coronary artery disease. *Annals of Internal Medicine* 110 (6): 456–69.

Is aerobic activity better than anaerobic activity for cardiac health?
Sesso H. D. et al. 2000. Physical activity and coronary heart disease in
    men: The Harvard alumni health study. American Heart Association.
    Circulation 102:975-980

Does heavy weight training increase muscle tension?
Siff, M. 2000. *Facts and fallacies of fitness.* Denver, CO: Mel Siff.

Do advanced athletes need to warm up before exercising?
Hale, J. 2007 *Knowledge and nonsense: The science of nutrition and
    exercise.* Winchester, KY: MaxCondition Publishing.
——. 2004. *MaxCondition.* Winchester, KY: MaxCondition Publishing.

Are sport-specific exercise programs beneficial?
Foran, B. 2001. *High-performance sports conditioning.* Champaign, IL:
    Human Kinetics.
Hale J. Designing sport-specific programs. MaxCondition. http://www
    .maxcondition.com/page.php?144 (accessed December 10, 2009).

Are slow training movements more effective than rapid movements?
Drechsler, A. 1998. *The weightlifting encyclopedia: A guide to world class
    performance.* Whitestone, NY: A Is A Communications.

Hale, J. 2007. *Knowledge and nonsense: The science of nutrition and exercise*. Winchester, KY. MaxCondition Publishing.
Siff, M. 2000. *Facts and fallacies of fitness*. Denver, CO: Mel Siff.

Is the motto "No pain, no gain" valid when working out?
Siff, M. 2000. *Facts and fallacies of fitness*. Denver, CO: Mel Siff.
——. 2000. *Supertraining*. Denver, CO: Mel Siff.

Should so-called dangerous exercises be avoided?
Siff, M. 2000. *Facts and fallacies of fitness*. Denver, CO: Mel Siff.
——. 2000. *Supertraining*. Denver, CO: Mel Siff.

Are strong abdominals the most important aspect of fitness?
Siff, M. 2000. *Facts and fallacies of fitness*. Denver, CO: Mel Siff
Zatsiorsky, V. 1995. *Science and practice of strength training*. Champaign, IL: Human Kinetics.

Are exercise machines safer than free weights?
Hale, J. 2003. Examining the rules of fitness. http://dolfzine.com/page596 .htm (site now discontinued).
——. Machine hoopla. MaxCondition. http://www.maxcondition.com/page .php?50 (accessed December 10, 2009).
Siff, M. 2000. *Facts and fallacies of fitness*. Denver, CO: Mel Siff.

Are strength and power the same thing?
Newton, H. 2002. *Explosive lifting for sports*. Champaign, IL: Human Kinetics.
Zatsiorsky, V. 1995. *Science and Practice of Strength Training*. Champaign IL: Human Kinetics.

Should women's fitness regimens be drastically different from men's?
Thornberry, A. Reaching the summit. http://www.maxcondition.com/page .php?77 (accessed December 10, 2009).
Siff, M. 2000. *Facts and fallacies of fitness*. Denver, CO: Mel Siff.

Should I Eat the Yolk?

Are certified fitness trainers highly qualified trainers?
Hale, J. 2004. *MaxCondition*. Winchester, KY: MaxCondition Publishing.
Siff, M. 2000. *Facts and fallacies of fitness*. Denver, CO: Mel Siff.

Does practice really "make perfect"?
Hale, J. 2004. *MaxCondition*. Winchester, KY: MaxCondition Publishing.
Siff, M. 2000. *Facts and fallacies of fitness*. Denver, CO: Mel Siff.

Is it necessary to exercise to lose weight?
Hale, J. Fat loss debate: Hale vs. Harmony. http://www.maxcondition.com/
    page.php?116 (accessed December 10, 2009).
Reuters. 2009. Obese Americans now outweigh the merely overweight.
    Reuters, January 9. http://www.reuters.com/article/domesticNews/
    idUSTRE50863H20090109 (accessed November 17, 2009).
Zelasko, C. J. 1995. Exercise for weight loss: What are the facts? *Journal of
    the American Dietetic Association* 95, no. 12 (December): 1414–17.

Are kettlebells more effective than barbells?
Hale, J. and D. Randolph. 2002. Kettlebells, how and why? MaxCondition
    http://www.maxcondition.com/page.php?33 (December 10, 2009).
——. 2007. *Knowledge and nonsense: The science of nutrition and exercise*.
    Winchester, KY: MaxCondition Publishing.

Does high-intensity exercise increase appetite?
Erdmann, J. et al. 2007. Plasma ghrelin levels during exercise—Effects
    of intensity and duration. *Regulatory Peptides* 143, no. 1–3
    (October):127–35.
Thompson, D. A. et al. 1988. Acute effects of exercise intensity on
    appetite in young men. *Medicine & Science in Sports & Exercise* 20,
    no. 3 (June): 222–27.

INDEX

A

Abdominal muscles, 98–99
  and exercise, 67–68, 82, 98–99
  and lifting belts, 69–70
  and sit-ups, 64–65
Adrenaline, 21
Adrenoreceptors, 62–63
Advanced Carbohydrate
  Classification System, 15
Aerobic exercise, 76–77, 112–13
  and fat loss, 71–72
  vs. anaerobic exercise, 91–92
  See also Exercise and exercise
    claims
Alcohol, and fat gain, 54
Alpha-receptors, 62–63

Alzheimer's disease, and ketogenic
  diets, 32
American Council of Science and
  Health, 59–60
Anaerobic vs. aerobic exercise,
  91–92
  See also Exercise and exercise
    claims
Antioxidants, 55–56
Appetite, and exercise, 106
Artificial sweeteners, 38–39,
  59–60
Aspartame (artificial sweetener),
  59–60
Athletes
  and aerobic exercises, 76–77
  and carbohydrates, 45, 46–48

and heavy weight training, 79

and protein, 34–35, 45

and warm-ups, 92–93

and water intake, 51–52

Atkins, Robert, 33–34

B

Back

exercises, 75–76, 83, 85

problems, 75–76

Barbells, 105–106

Beer gut, 54

Beta-carotene supplements, 55–56

Beta-receptors, 62–63

Blood flow, and stubborn body fat, 63

Blood pressure, and salt, 58

Blood sugar, and sugar alcohols, 45–46

Body fat, 62–64

and alcohol, 54

and ending weight training, 66

loss, 17–18, 71–72

Body measurements, 64–65, 108–109

Bone health, and high-protein diets, 25–26

Bottled water

safety, 15–16

taste, 16–17

Brain health

and low-carbohydrate diets, 32–33

C

Caffeinated beverages, and hydration, 51

Caffeine, 20–21, 51

Calcium

and high-protein diets, 25–26

and weight loss, 49–50

Calories, 111, 112

sources, 17–18

Carbohydrate loading, 46–48

Carbohydrates, 18–19

and athletes, 45, 46–48

and brain health, 32–33

excess, 48–49

and weight loss, 28–29, 33–34

Cardiac health, and exercise, 91–92

Cellulite, and exercise, 65–66

Certified fitness trainers, 102–103

Chest exercises, 82

Childhood epileptics, and ketogenic diets, 32

Children, and weight training, 68

Cholesterol levels, 37–38

Circuit training, and fitness, 77–78

Coffee
  and hydration, 51
  and insulin levels, 20–21
Corn syrup, 15, 60–61
Coronary heart disease (CHD)
  and eggs, 37–38
  and exercise, 91–92
  and high-protein diets,
    26–27
Cortisol blockers, and weight loss,
  24–25

D

Dairy products, 19, 113
  allergies and intolerance, 19,
    31–32
  and dieting, 31–32
  and weight loss, 49–50
De novo lipogenesis (DNL), 48–49
DeLorme method of sets/repetitions,
  73
Diabetes, 46
  and caffeine, 20
  and glycemic index, 28
  and sucralose, 39
Dietary cholesterol, 37–38
Dietary fat, 21
Dietary fiber, 42–43
Dietary supplements, 30–31, 55–56,
  109

Dieting and weight loss
  and calcium, 49–50
  and calories, 17–18, 111, 112
  and carbohydrates, 28–29, 33–34
  and cortisol blockers, 24–25
  and dairy products, 31–32
  and diets, 107–13
  and evening meals, 52–53
  and exercise, 104–105
  and food enjoyment, 20
  and fruit, 14–15
  and glycemic index, 28–29
  and grapefruit, 23–24
  and hypothyroidism, 22
  and insulin levels, 13–14
  and protein, 25–28, 110–11
  and snacking, 29–30
Downsize Me (film), 40
Dumbbells, 82, 111

E

Eating times
  frequency, 29–30
  and weight loss, 52–53
Egg yolks, 37–38
Endurance athletes
  and carbohydrates, 45
  and protein, 45
Equipment, 69–70, 72–73, 82, 84–85,
  99–101, 105–106, 111

Erythritol, and blood sugar, 45–46
Essential nutrients, 18–19
Exercise and exercise claims, 62–106,
    110, 112
    and appetite, 106
    dangerous, 97
    frequency, 110, 112
    injuries, 97
    intensity, 71–72
    repetition and practice,
        103–104
    speed, 95
    and stubborn body fat, 63
    and warm-ups, 92–93
    and weight loss, 104–105
    See also specific exercises
Exercise machines, 84–86, 99–101
    See also Equipment

F

Fat, in diet, 21
Fat gain, and alcohol, 54
Fat loss
    and aerobic exercise, 71–72
    and calories, 17–18
Fiber
    in diet, 42–43
    in fruit, 14
Fitness, and leanness, 86–87
Fitness trainers, 102–103

Flexibility
    and heavy weight training, 79
    and strength shoes, 73
Flouride levels, in water, 16
Food-combining theory, 22–23
Food log, 112
Food supplements, packaged, 109
Free weights, 99–101
Fructose, 14–15, 60–61
Fruit, 14–15

G

Ghrelin, 106
Glucose, 18–19
Glucose transporter type 1
    deficiency syndrome, and
    ketogenic diets, 32
Glycemic index (GI), 113
    and potatoes, 36–37
    and sugar alcohols, 46
    and weight loss, 28–29
"Good mornings" (back exercise), 83
Grapefruit
    and fat loss, 23–24
    and medications, 24

H

Hahnemann, Samuel, 57
Hanging leg raises, 67–68

Health and nutrition claims, 13–61
Heart problems. *See* Cardiac health;
   Coronary heart disease
Heavy weight training. *See* Weight
   training, heavy
High blood pressure, and salt, 58
High-fiber diets, 42–43
High-fructose corn syrup (HFCS), 15,
   60–61
High-intensity exercises, 71–72
High-protein diets, 25–28, 110–111
Hip flexors, and exercise, 67–68
Homeopathy, 56–57
Hormone receptors, 62–63
Hydration, 50–51. *See also* Water
Hypertension, and salt, 58
Hypothyroidism, and weight loss, 22

I

Injuries, causes, 97
Insulin levels, 13–14
   and coffee, 20–21
   and food combining, 23
   and fruit, 15
Isoflavones (soy), 43–44
Isomalt, 46

J

Junk food, 39–40

K

Ketogenic diets, and brain health,
   32–33
Kettlebells, 105–106
Kidneys, and high-protein diets,
   27–28
Knee extensions, 70
Knees
   exercises, 70
   locking during exercise, 74–75
   projection over toes, 81–82
   rehabilitation, 70

L

Lactitol, 46
Lactose intolerance, 19, 31–32
Leanness
   and fitness, 86–87
   and high-repetition weight
      training, 74
   and junk food, 39–40
Leg sleds, 85
Lifting belts, 69–70
Light weight training. *See* Weight
   training, light
Low-carbohydrate diets
   and brain health, 32–33
   and weight loss, 33–34
Low-fiber diets, 43

Lunges, 83–84
Lying leg press machines, 85

M

Maltitol, and blood sugar, 45–46
Mannitol, and blood sugar, 45–46
Meals, time of, 52–53
Meat and cheese diet, 25–28, 110–11
Medications, and grapefruit, 24
Memory disorders, and ketogenic
     diets, 32
Metabolism
     and muscle gain, 64
     and weight loss, 53–54
Milk products, 19, 113
     allergies and intolerance, 19,
          31–32
     and dieting, 31–32
     and weight loss, 49–50
Muscles
     bulk, 78, 80
     lengthening, 87
     soreness, 96
     tension, 92

N

Naringin, 23–24
National Council Against Health
     Fraud, 57

Natural Resources Defense Council
     (NRDC), 16
"No pain, no gain" concept, 96
Nutrition and health claims, 13–61

O

Obesity, 13–14
     and cortisol levels, 25
     and excess carbohydrates, 48–49
     and fruit, 14–15
     and high-fructose corn syrup,
          60–61
     and sugar, 35–36
Organic foods, 40–42
Osteoporosis, 25–26
Oxidation, 55–56
Oxygenated water, 42

P

Parkinson's disease, and ketogenic
     diets, 33
Performance-enhancing drugs,
     66–67
Phenylketonuria, 59–60
Pilates exercises, 87–89
Potatoes, 36–37
Power vs. strength, 95, 101
"Practice makes perfect" concept,
     103–104

Prescreen exercise testing, 90–91
Prone leg raises, 75–76
Prone trunk exercises, 75–76
Protein
    and athletes, 34–35, 45
    and bone health, 25–26
    and coronary heart disease,
        26–27
    and kidneys, 27–28
    RDA guidelines, 34–35
    and weight loss, 110–11
Pyruvate dehydrogenase complex
    deficiency, and ketogenic diets, 32

R

Rapid training movements, 95
Recommended Dietary Allowances
    (RDA) protein guidelines, 34–35
Relacore (cortisol blocker), and
    weight loss, 24–25
Repetitions, when exercising,
    73–74
Restenosis, and vitamin E, 56
Russet potatoes, 36–37

S

Safety, 81, 97, 99–101
Salt, 58
Satiety index, and potatoes, 37

Seated exercises, 69
Sets, when exercising, 73–74
Sex hormones, and dietary fat, 21
Sit-ups, 64–65
Snacking, and weight loss, 29–30
Sodium, 58
Sorbitol, 46
Soy products, 43–44
Spinal loading, 85
Spine stabilization, 82
Splenda (artificial sweetener),
    38–39
Sport-specific exercise programs,
    93–94
Sports science journals, and
    objectivity, 89
Sprinters, and heavy weight training,
    79
Squats, 83–84
    and knees, 70
Standing exercises, 69, 82
Steroids, 66–67, 78
Stomach, when exercising, 82. See
    also Abdominal muscles
Strength
    and muscular bulk, 78, 80
    and strength shoes, 72
    vs. power, 101
Strength shoes, 72–73
Stress tests, 90
Stubborn body fat, 62–64

Sucralose (artificial sweetener), 38–39

Sucrose, and obesity, 35–36

Sugars
  artificial, 38–39, 59–60
  in fruit, 15
  and obesity, 35–36
  types, 15

Supplements
  packaged food, 109
  vitamins and minerals, 30–31, 55–56

Suspended walking machines, 84–85

Sweet potatoes, 36–37

T

Tap water
  safety, 15–16
  taste, 16–17

Technique training, 103–104

Testosterone levels, and dietary fat, 21

Thyroid hormone, and weight loss, 22

Training and trainers, 102–103
  and professional body builders, 66–67, 78
  speed of movements, 95

Trunk exercises, 98–99

U

Undereating, 53–54

V

Vegetarian diet, and sex hormones, 21

Vitamin A supplements, 55–56

Vitamin C supplements, 55–56

Vitamin D, and high-protein diets, 25–26

Vitamin E supplements, 55–56

W

Waist measurement, and sit-ups, 64–65

Warm-ups, 92–93

Water
  and athletes, 51–52
  daily intake, 50–51
  intoxication, 50–51
  oxygenated, 42
  safety, 15–16
  taste, 16–17

Weaver, Chazz, 40

Weight gain, and food combining, 22–23

Weight loss. *See* Dieting and weight loss

Weight-loss programs, 107–13 *See also* Dieting and weight loss
Weight training, 111
  and children, 68
  equipment, 69–70, 72–73, 82, 84–85, 99–101, 105–106, 111
  heavy, 78–79, 81, 92
  high repetition, 74
  light, 81
  safety, 81, 97, 99–101
  vs. Pilates, 88–89
White potatoes, 36–37
Women
  fitness regimens, 102
  and heavy weight training, 78
Workout schedules, 110, 112

X

Xylitol, 46

Y

Yohimbe, and stubborn body fat, 63–64
Yolks, 37–38

Other Ulysses Press Books

7 WEEKS TO 100 PUSH-UPS: STRENGTHEN AND SCULPT YOUR ARMS, ABS, CHEST, BACK AND GLUTES BY TRAINING TO DO 100 CONSECUTIVE PUSH-UPS
Steve Speirs, $14.95
This book is the ultimate program to train the body to go from just one push-up to 100 consecutive reps in under two months—sculpting muscles in the chest, abs, back, glutes and arms without a single piece of unwieldy equipment.

101 HEALTHIEST FOODS: A QUICK AND EASY GUIDE TO THE FRUITS, VEGETABLES, CARBS AND PROTEINS THAT CAN SAVE YOUR LIFE
Dr. Joanna McMillan Price and Judy Davie, $14.95
A handy and easy-to-use guide that identifies the 101 healthiest foods in the world, decribing the life-saving nutritional value for each foods plus details why they are the best choice within their food group.

THE ANATOMY OF MARTIAL ARTS: AN ILLUSTRATED GUIDE TO THE MUSCLES USED FOR EACH STRIKE, KICK, AND THROW
Lily Chou and Norman Link, $16.95
The perfect training supplement for martial artists, this book's detailed anatomical drawings show exactly what is happening inside the body while it's performing a physical movement.

BLACK BELT KRAV MAGA: ELITE TECHNIQUES OF THE WORLD'S MOST POWERFUL COMBAT SYSTEM
Darren Levine & Ryan Hoover, $15.95
For the first time, *Black Belt Krav Maga* teaches and illustrates the discipline's most lethal fighting and self-defense moves in book format.

COMPLETE KRAV MAGA: THE ULTIMATE GUIDE TO OVER 230 SELF-DEFENSE AND COMBATIVE TECHNIQUES
Darren Levine & John Whitman, $21.95
Clearly written and extensively illustrated, *Complete Krav Maga* details every aspect of this easy-to-learn yet highly effective system, including hand-to-hand combat moves and weapons defense techniques.

CORPS STRENGTH: A MARINE MASTER GUNNERY SERGEANT'S PROGRAM
FOR ELITE FITNESS
MGySgt. Paul J. Roarke, $14.95
Renowned for its rigorous fitness training, the Marine Corps requires every member
to be physically fit, regardless of age, grade, or duty assignment. *Corps Strength*
applies the same techniques used to develop and maintain each Marine's combat
readiness to a day-to-day program for top-level fitness.

THE EASY GL DIET HANDBOOK: LOSE WEIGHT WITH THE REVOLUTIONARY GLYCEMIC
LOAD PROGRAM
Dr. Fedon Alexander Lindberg, $10.00
Using these more accurate and sensible GL scores, *The Easy GL Diet Handbook*
offers a plan for healthy weight loss and reduced risk of diabetes that's easier to
follow. It also includes numerous foods that the Atkins, South Beach, and GI diets
wrongly consider "off-limits."

THE GI MEDITERRANEAN DIET: THE GLYCEMIC INDEX-BASED LIFE-SAVING DIET OF
THE GREEKS
Dr. Fedon Alexander Lindberg, $14.95
Mediterranean cuisine and GI dieting are a proven match made in culinary heaven.
This book shows readers how the Old World's most celebrated foods can keep you
lean, young and living a longer and healthier life.

TOTAL HEART RATE TRAINING: CUSTOMIZE AND MAXIMIZE YOUR WORKOUT USING
A HEART RATE MONITOR
Joe Friel, $15.95
Shows anyone participating in aerobic sports, from novice to expert, how to
increase the effectiveness of his or her workout by utilizing a heart rate monitor.

*To order these books call 800-377-2542 or 510-601-8301, fax 510-601-8307, e-mail
ulysses@ulyssespress.com, or write to Ulysses Press, P.O. Box 3440, Berkeley, CA
94703. All retail orders are shipped free of charge. California residents must include
sales tax. Allow two to three weeks for delivery.*

ABOUT THE AUTHOR

JAMIE HALE is sports-conditioning coach who was inducted into the World Marital Arts Hall of Fame in recognition of his conditioning work with competitive martial artists. In 2008 Jamie's gym, Total Body Fitness, which he owned and operated for eleven years, was featured in *Men's Health* as one of the top-30 training facilities in the U.S. He is considered by most in the industry as a specialist in agility and comprehensive fitness training. Jamie's scientific approach and critical-thinking ability has earned him the nicknames "The Practical Scientist" and "The Fitness Skeptic." He has written for *Men's Health*, *MMA Sports Magazine*, *Planet Muscle*, *Mind and Muscle* magazine, *Speed Strength*, and *Sport Athlete*.